UPDATING LIFE AND DEATH

L. E. Rothstein

U. mass. - Amherst

Dept. of Poli. Sci.

UPDATING
LIFE and DEATH

Essays in Ethics and Medicine

Edited by Donald R. Cutler

Beacon Press   Boston

CONTENTS

INTRODUCTION

by Donald R. Cutler

TWO FACTORS might well lead the ordinary reflective person to assume that our society is generating a voluminous literature concerned with ethics and medicine. It is not. One might expect, for example, a more extensive literature on medical ethics than is being published about the ethics of war or the ethics of affluence, scarcity, and hunger.

The first factor consists of the ubiquity of the issues and themes of medical ethics. The practice of medicine and medical research touches virtually all of us who have more than enough to eat and who, given the propensity of Americans to resolve their international conflicts on foreign soil, have limited expectations of being touched directly by warfare. Most of us are familiar, however, with critical medical decisions on which have rested the welfare — if not in fact the continuance of life itself — of ourselves or our closest kin.

Professional ethicists may be more self-conscious than non-ethicists of the second factor, but the factor itself is relevant to anyone who thinks about the justice and meaning of how he lives and what he does. The dilemmas of medical practice are interesting in that the boundaries of the practical situations can be comparatively clearly defined; within these boundaries, the several technical, professional, social, and cultural factors can be distinguished rather easily.

Consider briefly the dimensions of an episode which occurred as this volume was being edited for publication. Americans were informed of the first successful *im*plantation of an artificial heart in a human being. This implantation was performed in the absence of a donated heart for *trans*plantation. Urgent appeals for an organic heart were broadcast, and the patient himself revealed some of the mythology implicit in the situation by declaring that he wished to be a man with a real heart ("real" hearts in this case being defined as organs composed of human tissue).

In Massachusetts, the family of a comatose woman afflicted with irreparable brain damage responded to the appeal from Texas and made the decision to donate in behalf of the comatose woman. The donor was flown to Texas in a dramatic flight during which her heart was reported to have stopped beating at least once and to have been revived by emergency techniques. The implanted heart was replaced with a transplanted heart after extraordinary techniques to keep the donor's heart functioning in her body had been withdrawn.

Ironically, the donee lived longer with the implanted artificial heart than with the transplanted tissue heart. After his death arguments were published about the wisdom of the *im*plantation and the extent to which federal guidelines had been followed regarding the application of research funded in part by the government. A concurrent controversy centered on the matter of who should properly claim credit for the invention of the artificial heart; the vanity of medical practice surfaced temporarily through the ordinary bland professional veneer. The technology, politics, economics, and social psychology of medical innovation are all transparent in this episode; when that is the case ethical reflection has a suitable context for careful formulation.

One finds it easy to sympathize with the ethicist on Vietnam who must compensate for uneven and incomplete reporting, classified information, deliberate obscuring of actual policy, and the real but tantalizingly vague outlines of a "military-industrial complex." Why, however, if medicine touches us all and deeply and if the cluster of factors relevant to ethical reflection is unusually available, have we not written and published more than now exists in print?

Perhaps it is that the subject is too close to our life interests. It may be less troubling to ponder the justice of a war over there, the administration of which pleased 46 per cent of us last month and 51 per cent this month. We do, it is true, prefer issues which can be reduced to a single graphic image: the body of a donor en route to Texas, the starving child in Biafra, the cops in Chicago.

But we also prefer those issues to be remote so that we can experience sympathy, not direct confrontation. To the extent we have ourselves experienced the situations out of which medical ethics are formulated, we are apt to have experienced them in relation to pain, guilt, anxiety, loss, and trauma — episodes we are in part motivated to repress, not to rationalize and interpret.

Participation in the development of medical ethics requires a predisposition to acknowledge a good deal of paradox, irony, and conflict. The society willing to underwrite techniques costing scores of thousands of dollars to extend the life of a single patient is simultaneously concerned with overpopulation, the justifiable circumstances for abortion, and the merits of voluntary and involuntary euthanasia. The ethicist has to rationalize wise rules and insights for a society in which, simultaneously, healthy persons literally offer their hearts to a patient desperate for a transplant and research physicians conduct experimentation involving pain and/or danger without informed consent on the part of the patient-subject.

The purpose of *Updating Life and Death* is to introduce the reader to a number of levels of inquiry germane to the whole field of ethics and medicine. The several contributions were not written in deliberate collaboration, and each therefore deserves to be read as a multifaceted expression of the writer's preoccupations. Most of the essays were commissioned specifically for *The Religious Situation: 1968* or *The Religious Situation: 1969,* however, with the expectation that a paperback edition would eventually permit a merger of the material. The reader may therefore wish to know something of what the editor had in mind.

The environment in which critical medical decisions are typically made is perceived by the ordinary man to be dominated by professionalism and technology. Joseph Fletcher corrects this perception in "Our Shameful Waste of Human Tissue" by analyzing the extent to which medical decisions are influenced by images and conceptions we hold about the body and its destiny. These images and conceptions are projected in religious doctrine and practice, legal structures, and other cultural expressions. The heart, therefore, is not just a circulatory pump; it is "the seat of the soul, the source of courage." When it develops techniques for swapping hearts, medical-technological progress has to contend with the mythology of the body as much as with surgical techniques or methods to inhibit organ-rejection.

Fletcher is concerned principally with the ethics of beliefs and attitudes which inhibit potential donors and their kin from making the decisions of life-or-death consequence for donees. Dr. M. H. Pappworth, in "Ethical Issues in Experimental Medicine," raises the advantages and protections of nontechnological and nonprofessional factors. Appalled, as a physician, by the extent of medical experimentation without need or consent, he concludes that "The Churches, the Law, and Parliament must express their opinions collectively and state how much further they are prepared to allow the medical profession to take risks with human lives in order to achieve possible advances in knowledge."

The development of respirators and heart-lung machines has made us more aware than we were of the boundary at which new therapeutic techniques challenge the adequacy of symbols by which we define health and illness, life and death. Any revision of that symbolism has implications for ethics. Two contributions to this volume are addressed to this problem of revised symbolism, and from interestingly different perspectives.

Machines can now sustain the vital organ functions of some patients believed to be irreversibly comatose. The machines can keep "alive" persons whose hearts and lungs would otherwise cease to function — cease to function perhaps in circumstances which would prevent transplantation of organs from the comatose patient to waiting donees. The machines therefore make transplants more feasible; but how does one rationalize when and why one turns off the machine for humane, economic, or transplant reasons.

The *Ad Hoc* Committee of the Harvard Medical School to Examine the Definition of Brain Death (chaired by Dr. Henry K. Beecher) speaks from the perspective of a group most of whom are involved in medical research. Conditions for transplants which will not abuse donors' interests are very much in the forefront of their suggestions. Paul Ramsey, in "On Updating Death," looks at the same questions from an equally penetrating but quite different point of departure:

> I shall argue . . . that there is sufficient need and sufficient reason in the dying or dead patient's own care, and that of his family, for clarifying or revising our understanding of death. The needs of potential recipients of organs need not and should not be brought into view even as adjunct considerations [p. 41].

In the first four chapters of this volume the reader will encounter four distinguishably different approaches to the ethics of organ transplants. Discussions of ethics flourish when contending views are presented in juxtaposition. The adequacy of the climate of ethical reflection can be increased also by an analysis which itself tries to describe a range of positions.

A debate on the ethics of abortion has been evoking headlines for the past few years; the debate has raged in legislatures, churches, classrooms, and in the mass media. Seldom has the controversy been controlled or sustained enough for the observer or participant to discern the fundamental line of argumentation on each of the several sides of the debate. In the fifth chapter, Ralph B. Potter, Jr., unravels the debate; his analysis is a model of the kind of overview one would like to have available for every major issue of applied ethics. In the following chapter Arthur Dyck has contributed a crosscultural analysis of the population crisis. His data make clear the extent to which varieties of culture and religion predispose us to construct varieties of attitudes and policies toward common problems.

The abortion debate is a principal factor in the background of Herbert Richardson's "What Is The Value of Life?" Over time, and in ways that vary from society to society and era to era (and in fact within a personality and its own experience or life history), men extrapolate from the accumulation of experience a sense of what they value. Once identified, a value then becomes an ideal reality of a sort that one may try to realize deliberately in personal or social life. Richardson shows how the difficult issues of ethics and medicine are apt to involve conflict between values we espouse. But value conflict appears to some extent to be a prerequisite for the evolution of the better integration of old values and the conception of new values.

Few values in our society evoke more lip service than "the sanctity of life." Daniel Callahan, in the eighth chapter, submits the critical value of sanctity to very detailed analysis, indicating how difficult it is to justify values philosophically; the inherent abstraction and ambiguity of the phraseology of values imperils the opportunity even for men of good will to agree on the literal meaning of the sanctity of life. The principle of the sanctity of life does, however, stand in relation to the "lower-level" systems of rules, and when the principle is shared by men of common conviction life is in fact sanctified in the decisions men make. Julian Pleasants, Dr. Henry K. Beecher, and James Gustafson present critiques of Callahan's essay, to which Callahan writes a concluding response.

The final chapter is addressed to a contemporary controversy among technologists, ecologists, and philosophers. From whence should the vision evolve for the society we are bringing into existence? Are the fundamental decisions about updating life and death responsible finally to technology or to ecology? New medical developments depend mainly on technology, and worldviews are available now in predominantly technological form and language. Frederick Elder argues the wisdom of grounding visions and plans in ecological terms and of restoring biocentric factors to parity with anthropocentric factors.

The perceived implication of a volume stressing varieties of advice and ranging from specific medical techniques to the most abstract reflection might be to discourage the reader from believing that the updating of life and death can be accomplished charitably and constructively. The intent of the volume, however, is in the opposite direction. In blindness and ignorance we are most apt to destroy ourselves, especially when we have developed more and more remarkable technological facilities. Wise decisions require insight at all the levels presented here. Participation in this multilevel debate is available to every man.

UPDATING LIFE AND DEATH

1. OUR SHAMEFUL WASTE OF HUMAN TISSUE: AN ETHICAL PROBLEM FOR THE LIVING AND THE DEAD

by Joseph Fletcher

WE HAVE entered a new era medically, and therefore culturally — i.e., morally and ideologically. There are many highly portentous "breakthroughs" in modern medicine but the one under scrutiny here we can call the Spare Parts Program.

Surgery and medicine, in partnership with technology, can *transplant* tissue by a graft from one person to another, such as skin or bone and organs like a liver or a heart, and from one part to another in the same person, such as blood vessels or cartilage. They can *implant* artificial materials and machines — e.g., synthetic arteries and electronic cardiac pacemakers. And they can *supplant* tissue — for example, with synthetic and plastic heart valves, or with kidney machines which can carry on the work of hemodialysis without the natural organ altogether. A lot of this spare parts or "cyborg" medicine is only in an early stage of success, but it is here [6].

In World War II they called it "cannibalizing" when they put together parts of damaged lorries to make up whole ones. This kind of reconstruction is now an accomplished part of medicine [8]. Not very long ago we found a measure of gallow's humor in saying that a dead body or cadaver was worth about 87 cents — for its residual chemicals. But now a body has become very valuable — indeed, supremely precious — in terms of its lifesaving values.

Too much of the time when we speak of our era as a technological one we have only discerned its character. We haven't really grasped it yet. In the midst of knowledge and power explosions it is easy to let the present turn a corner into the future when we are looking the other way; then we get left too far behind. As Marshall McLuhan says, we live in a "rear-view mirror." We are not even as quick as Alice in her looking glass. We think of new things retrospectively, speaking of radios as "wirelesses" and autos as "horseless carriages" and trains as "iron horses" and refrigerators as "ice boxes" and cinematography as "moving pictures."

As we shall see, we are caught in something of this same lag with respect to medicine, and the result is that we are being prodigally wasteful in our funerary practices and stupidly selfish in our use of vital organs while we live and even more so when we die. It may not be too much to say that very often so-called reverent or pious death ceremonies, solemn "rites of passage" in the language of Van Gennep and the anthropologists, are nothing more than acts of callous indifference, and that our dying nowadays (80% of it in hospitals, not at home) is followed through in complete and selfish disregard of the health and even survival needs of the living. What follows will be an explication of this charge.

THE PROBLEM — THE ISSUE

The problem arises because medicine needs more "spare parts" for transplantation than it can find, and the issue is a cultural-ethical one — ought we not to donate the human parts and tissue needed to save or enhance lives, and to give social reinforcement to such donations, whether the donors are well or near to dying? Emerson (in *Gifts*) said, "The only gift is a portion of thyself." He spoke more truly than he knew; we can take him far more literally than he ever imagined.

In New York City, to take just one major urban community, there are always from fifty to a hundred victims of kidney disease on chronic dialysis (periodic blood-cleansing by a machine *ex corpo*), waiting in line for a new kidney from either a living donor who has volunteered to share one kidney or from a cadaver, i.e., the body of another patient who willed his kidneys for extraction and transplant after death. In cases of renal failure alone, 7,644 patients died in the United States in 1963. In the same year there were 10,600 kidneys available from patients dying of subarachnoid hemorrhage, a fairly abrupt death which leaves the kidneys in a normal condition. Even after ruling some out as diseased or incompatible there would have been more than enough kidneys to meet the need [4].

Given good surgical-medical logistics, and getting the moral-religious blocks out of the way, death or prolonged dialysis for lack of spare kidneys would be close to ended. It has been estimated that 14,000 to 15,000 kidneys per year could be made available from people dying of brain damage in other forms. In the same year (1963) 4,000 livers were needed, which the same 5,300 hemorrhage victims could have supplied. But in fact, nearly all of these kidney patients died while vital organs were being burned up in cremation or buried to rot in the ground. In 1967 only 700 renal transplants were performed because donors are so hard to enlist. There are already recorded instances of flat refusals to allow hearts to be transplanted from prospective donors, in a field of spare-parts medicine which has only had a year of practice in the operating theatre. (A quick glance at *Index Medicus* will show how extraordinarily little is published about cadavers, tissue donation, and organ procurement.)

The resistance to this new dimension of man's struggle against disease and death comes mainly from deep-seated feelings about the body. The sense of identity and recognition is largely somatic, especially for the simple-minded. Even though we suffer when we lose a part of our own flesh and bone we don't lose our self-recognition; we know who we are no matter how maimed we may be. It is, therefore, probably somewhat easier psychologically to volunteer a part of one's self than it is for family or friends to dispose of one's body on their own initiative. There are many situations in which kidneys, for example, have been promised by a donor patient, but nevertheless after death the family refuse to allow it. It seems somehow to them to be destroying or hurting or degrading those who have "passed on." Add to this image-making the powerful guilt components in grief reactions, familiar to us all, and we have no great difficulty in understanding (though not necessarily condoning) such "blocks" in the way of ethical responsibility. (The legal position is often so unclear and the sensibilities so poignant that hospital officials and physicians have usually bowed to this obstructionism, often at the expense of the recipient patient's life.)

The popular tendency has always been to combine vitalistic and organismic notions in the feeling that *life* somehow depends on organic unity and integrity, and that therefore personal identity or the *soul* does too. This popular sentiment is never made up of philosophical rhetoric. Indeed, its typical language-form is religious instead, commonly in terms of a belief in or longing for survival after death. Few if any religious doctrines of eternal life and personal survival are so formulated theologically that the person to be "saved" is essentially corporeal, but the hunch-feeling persists that the *body* is sacrosanct; it is a form of religious materialism or physicalism [see 14]. Western piety and folkways have commonly lost sight of the warnings against this by Aristotle when he first gave a full-dress defense of the notion in *The Soul* and in *The Generation of Animals* as far back as the middle of the fourth century B.C. Christians, for example, forget or ignore Saint Paul's emphatic declaration, "It is sown a physical body, it is raised a spiritual body" [3].

It has been a long time since very many people explicitly and consciously believed in the "resurrection of the body" in a kind of naive, non-Pauline conception of the "raised body" as a physical or material levitation or ascension. But just beneath the surface many people still *feel* that to lose a limb or an organ or a cornea is to enter "whatever comes next" halt, maimed and blind. In the period from the first to the sixth century many, indeed the majority of Christians, believed that the "saved" would, in duplication of Jesus' resurrection and ascension, rise from the grave and go "up" into eternal life — usually *en masse* at the last trump. In spite of the word games played rather skillfully by theologians to keep "body" from being understood in the flesh sense, it has been so taken and in some sects still is [see 2:208–226 for a recent sample of theological skill].

In modern times we have seen a considerable decline of explicit belief in an afterlife. Among the Semitic religions this has not much troubled Judaism, which is relatively unmetaphysical and without any developed speculation about personal survival after death, but it has changed the focus of Christian and Moslem attitudes toward a more this-worldly concern. By a happy twist, when we recall the history of classical and orthodox beliefs, this loss of faith in "heaven" and "the next world" tends to enhance appreciation of human life and values. And the modern man's understanding of soul and identity, cut loose from an earnest faith in immortality, *should* logically free people from the feeling that their real selves depend upon their keeping their bodies intact for the future life beyond the grave. Combined with theological reinterpretations of "body," this disappearance of eternity orientation should make it easier to overcome fearful and defensive objections to donating spare parts.

MUTILATION

The body taboo adversely affects not only transplants but medical knowledge and education. People not only fail or refuse to offer their organs to transplant surgery, they also withhold them from the medical schools. And even from autopsy. We all know the story of the "resurrectionists" or body snatchers in the early nineteenth century, who came into being because anatomists could not legally get bodies for dissection, and how they continued their grotesque robberies of graves until somewhat more enlightened laws allowed unclaimed bodies from prisons and poorhouses to go to medical schools instead of potter's fields. (Statute law reflects the intelligence and morality of the lawmakers and, in a democracy, of the people in general.) The problem of supply is very, very far from solved.

In 1519 Pope Leo X denied Leonardo da Vinci admission to a Rome hospital to study anatomy because he had once engaged in dissection. It was not until 1737 that Benedict XIV gave official papal approval of it, which was repeated recently by Pius XII in an allocution to eye specialists in May, 1956. But to this day rabbis and mullahs are divided in their opinions.

Even today, we in the West are not too far advanced from the state of mind in which five people were killed in a riot in April, 1788, following a mob burning of the Hospital Society's building at Reed and Duane Streets in downtown New York because it housed an anatomy collection. They wanted "no fooling with human bodies," and their attitude hangs on.

In 1964, 7,400 cadavers were needed for optimum instruction in American medical schools, but outside of 2,000 unclaimed bodies available from morgues or other public agencies there were only 600 available by bequest — in the whole of the United States [38]. These served only one-third of the need. Welfare benefits for the aged or indigent, since the Second World War, have greatly reduced the supply from the poor-dead.

In some cities medical education alleviates the problem of scarcity by sharing. For example, in Boston the three major medical schools (Harvard, Tufts, and Boston University) maintain a Coordinator of Anatomical Material. This helps considerably. On the encouraging side, incidentally, there is a discernible increase in the number of *donated* bodies, while the supply of unclaimed bodies has dropped off. And in Boston the number of young people making a testamentary disposition of their bodies for dissection or transplant increases relatively, and those given only at the last minute, in terminal illness, decreases relatively. (To summarize the 1961–1966 figures for the Boston schools: *willed* bodies increased to five times as many as were received from 1956–1961 (from 68 to 326); *unclaimed* bodies decreased (from 670 to 562); and there were 150 *more* received during the later period.)

When a choice has to be made between dissection for study or autopsy for diagnosis, the schools give way — on the ground, reasonable enough, that diagnostic or medico-legal requirements come first. Even here, in autopsy procedure, the body taboo constantly undermines moral obligation and responsibility to society. While 1.8 million Americans die each year — four-fifths of them in hospitals, only one-fifth in homes — *only one in six* is autopsied in spite of medical insistence on it for the sake of critical and research inquiry. (The better the hospital the more autopsies are done. In the Massachusetts General Hospital, for instance, 70% of the dead are autopsied. Pathologists and their staffs have an important role in good medicine.)

The religious hurdles which continue to undermine ethical concern and modern humanitarianism were shown in April, 1967, by an outbreak of Orthodox Jews attacking the Knesset and government. In Tel Aviv and Jerusalem they demonstrated in protest against autopsy.

[This was tied to Talmudic law requiring that corpses be buried on the day of death, a rule which has run into much conflict with coroners' proceedings because of the hasty interment. The moral law also forbids a priest (kohen) or his descendants to come within four cubits of a cadaver, or to be under the same roof with one [16:236–241].]

Some 358 religious leaders, including the two chief rabbis, called for the repeal of a 1953 law which allowed autopsies when three physicians certified a need to determine the cause of death. Judges in rabbinical courts asked synagogues to add to the Yom Kippur liturgy, "Our Father, our King, repel the evil of autopsies." People began refusing to enter hospitals, afraid their bodies would be "violated" if they died.

Rigid and orthodox Jewish religious law forbids mutilation, except if it is necessary in order to save the patient's life, or possibly for investigation in a mysterious plague [see 18:96–98]. This is a serious obstruction to transplant medicine, donations to eye banks, and the like.

[Rabbi Joseph B. Soloveitchik, a distinguished Orthodox scholar, has said that the "halachic community" (the people of the law) find no moral questions about transplants *inter vivos* if there is no more than a statistical risk for the donor, and that the Talmudic position allows for cadaveric transplants too [35].]

The rabbinate has approved of organ transplants on the principle of "pikuakh nefesh," which permits breaking moral laws if life is in danger. The Ashkenazic Chief Rabbi in Israel declared (August, 1968) that transplants are allowed to save living patients but organs may not be stored. Roman Catholic moral philosophy took much the same position until quite recently. (As we often find in these matters of specific or concrete moral questions, there is no Protestant discussion on surgery, autopsy, and other mutilative procedures — not even on the ethics of transplant donation.) In just the past five years, under the pressure of spare-parts medicine as it has jumped forward, we have seen a marked and welcome change in Catholic moral theology. As recently as May, 1956, nevertheless, Pius XII expressed a papal disapproval of any attempt to offer an ethical justification for *inter vivos* transplants, from one living person to another, or for mutilations of any kind for any reason at all except to save the patient's life or health. But ten years later the weight of theological opinion was and is against Pope Pius. (It is interesting to compare the even development of Catholic opinion on this question to the ups and downs of the contraception controversy — especially in the light of Paul VI's reaction against "artificial" birth control, in July, 1968 [see pp 670–691].)

CONCERN FOR OTHERS: A RELUCTANT VIRTUE

In 1944 Fr. B. J. Cunningham published his *Morality of Organic Transplantation*, the first full-dress Catholic moral defense of the procedure [5; 25]. It fluttered the dovecotes. A long-standing principle of Catholic moral theology, the principle of totality, holds that (as Aquinas put it) the whole is more important than its parts, and therefore a *diseased* part may be sacrificed to save the health or life of the whole body [21]. But does this mean that one may only undergo organ excision (mutilation) for one's own sake, not for another's? For example, is it permissible in cases of prefrontal lobotomy or appendectomy, but not of donor nephrectomy or donor ovariectomy? The answer had been, for a long time, a clear "Yes."

Things began moving in this century. In 1899–1900 H. Noldin said that a voluntary offer of any tissue would be a "violation of the Fifth Commandment" and "intrinsically unlawful" [37:328n]. But in 1923 A. Vermeersch could, to the contrary, say it would be "licit and commendable, though not of obligation" — i.e., justifiable on grounds of charity and the unity of mankind, but not required in conscience [37:323n]. However, the question was as yet so little pressing that both of these opposed opinions were given in footnotes. Father Cunningham's treatise opened it fully, a whole decade before kidney transplants started on an important scale.

The issue was over invasion of a person's totality or bodily integrity. It did not affect post mortem mutilations. As McFadden points out, there is no ethical objection to cremation, dissection, autopsy, embalming, or bone banks contributed to *after* death [26:265–266]. Canon law allows hospitals to dispose non-ceremonially of amputated limbs, excised organs, and so on, although burial in "holy ground" is preferred. Nor is there any moral objection, then, to organ transplants post mortem or cadaveric; the objection only arises with ante mortem or *inter vivos* donations.

In the whole matter of transplants, however, Cunningham had rested the case for them on a theory of radical solidarism, or the oneness of human beings as the family of God. He reasoned from this base that to give an ovary or testicle (or graft therefrom, as in the Voronoff procedure), or to give a kidney or an eye or any other paired organ, is not only an act of charity or loving concern but actually "selfish" or self-serving in the sense that the recipient is only the other self, an alter ego. It was this thesis in moral theology, and its conclusion, which Pius XII rejected in 1956.

Once the papal view had been published doubt and disagreement began to be expressed. The official opinion amounted to this: that one may morally save his own life or health but not his neighbor's! Healy interprets Pius to have meant that "mutilation is licit only when necessary for preserving the health of the whole body" — i.e., the individual's own body [17:122]. This was practically the language also of Pius XI, in his encyclical *Casti Connubii*, 1930. McFadden puts it in other words, that Pius meant one may not deliberately submit to mutilation "to help some other person or to assist Society" [26:267].

As the Jesuit moralist Gerald Kelly once said, it may "come as a surprise" to hear that it is wrong when donors "have as their purpose the helping of others" — in short, that it is wrong to be a *living* donor [20:246]. Father Kelly could not accept it. Nor can most Catholic theologians of this day. It is recognized that to give a singular organ such as the heart is suicide, and no Catholic moralist is willing (as yet) to defend that much sacrifice. But sharing paired organs such as a kidney is another matter. McFadden, for one, defends donations *inter vivos* on the grounds that the principle of totality calls for *functional* integrity, not mere anatomical integrity. On this view we may rightly remove a healthy appendix because it has no vital function or purpose, and we may give up a kidney because one (or even a third of one) might be enough to preserve renal function. Only if donor nephrectomies are shown to impair a necessary function are they to be declared illicit. Healy takes the same stand, speaking of "substantial" integrity or totality, but meaning functional.

[In 1953 the Central Conference of American Rabbis received a report from its committee on responsa saying that "the dismemberment of a human body after death is not regarded as a mutilation, if other lives, now imperiled or seriously impaired, might be rescued" — but this applies only to autopsy, not to ante mortem gifts of organs or other tissue. Nor does it provide for medical school use [42:153]. To date the Conference has issued no ethical approval of spare-parts medicine. It seems, strangely enough, that unlike all other religions, Judaism in early times was unopposed to dissection, and its rabbinical formulations only later became unfavorable [18:136].]

JOSEPH FLETCHER · *Our Shameful Waste of Human Tissue*

Running any risk entailed, according to Healy, is legitimate for due reason.

There is, on this basis, little or no reason to question the morality of cadaveric transplants, or of giving one's organs for that purpose by ante mortem testament. As J. J. Lynch, S.J., sees it, there are no objections *per se* to a cadaveric transplant, although there might be objections *per accidens* — i.e., in a particular situation. He asks only that three rational preconditions be satisfied: 1) it is a necessary means of last resort, 2) there is a reasonable hope of substantial benefit, and 3) the medical and surgical team are competent [24]. This applies also to kidneys, livers, endocrines, lungs, corneas, skin, bones, blood vessels — to all organs paired or unpaired, and to all kinds of human tissue. Our problem is not so much with the theologians as with inhibited or indifferent rank-and-file clergy and doctors who either do not know these things or do not care or will not bother to think about them or teach and lead the people they profess to serve.

The trap into which religious ethicists fall is, of course, their legalism. They adumbrate "principles" or universals as first premises for their syllogistic reasoning, and then as empirical experience undermines their generalizations and situations change the "context" in which human values are to be served, they are paralyzed by these first premises — which they usually suppose to have some sort of divine authority. As Henry D. Aiken and others have pointed out, the more primitive or religious a culture or tradition is the more legalistic or rigid its morality, and the more mature and sophisticated it is the more elastic and situational its morality [1:116–127]. Anthropology has provided convincing data to support this.

It is often said in medical circles that these ethical problems are questions without answers. This is true in the sense that there are no completely reliable generalizations of a normative kind to dictate or pre-decide what we ought to do. We cannot universalize or make absolute right and wrong, however loyal we may be to such values as human well-being and response to need. Nevertheless, there *are* answers in the sense of responsible and reasonable decisions in particular cases, and this — along with the insights we gain by good question-asking — is all we can or need to have. This is medical responsibility.

The term "responsibility" calls for one comment before we pass on to a brief account of what is going on in spare-parts medicine. Especially in medicine the term should not be given a merely juridical or legal sense, but this is true in ethical discourse too. The common notion is that it means answerability — the willingness or ability to be called to account, to stand before an authority or nemesis (usually judging our acts according to preset rules). But the term is better and more correctly understood as response, the ability and willingness to respond to human need, to answer a call for help in a concrete and particular situation. Therefore the phrase "moral responsibility" is essentially redundant, since to be moral or act morally is to be responsive to people. Morality *is* responsibility. And the response factor is the key [see 10; 13:231–241].

PRESENT PRACTICE

Most of the experience in organ transplantation to date has come from kidney dialysis and replacement. It got off to a good start in 1954 with a transplant done by Dr. Murray, Dr. Merrill, and Dr. Harrison at Peter Bent Brigham Hospital in Boston [30]. Up to that time the only spare-parts surgery, except for corneas, had been structural (e.g., bone and cartilage) or cosmetic (e.g., skin and hair), but now it had reached the *functional* level, the level of vital life-or-death functions.

At first the kidneys were isografts, i.e., from related donors *inter vivos*. In fact, because of the problem of rejection or "immune reaction," twins were the most promising donors and recipients. But gradually allografts (from unrelated donors) have been successful as immunosuppressive methods have improved, to the point that by now there is a much higher rate of success, coming close to equal. Survival data on 1,178 transplants (through 1966) yield estimates of 65% survival for related donors and of

39% for unrelated — a year following the operation [29]. These data come from first and second transplants in 63 hospitals in 19 counties, and show that *kidneys from living donors*, compared to cadaver kidneys, require fewer dialyses prior to transplantation, fail less often to "start," have fewer rejection crises, and only half as many have to be rehospitalized. The longest surviving renal allograft recipient has been in normal health for over eight years [28].

Helped by surgical experience, compatibility testing, and better immunosuppression, transplantation has moved from twin donors to related donors to unrelated donors and from living to cadaveric transfers. Cadaveric transplants from unrelated donors allow for *two* kidneys, not just one. At Mt. Sinai Hospital in New York recently a man died of brain disease; one of his kidneys went to a 16-year-old boy and one went to a 48-year-old woman. A cadaver-pancreas has been stitched to the recipient's old and failing one; if it rejects they can snip it off and all is as before. An auto fatality in 1968 in São Paulo, Brazil, yielded a heart to one patient and a kidney to another; following a suicide in the same city, the heart and both kidneys and the pancreas were transplanted. The same "mix" was performed in Houston, Texas, except that a lung rather than the pancreas was used.

It is reasonable to see a further advance in the use of animal organs, i.e., xenografts, but that is in the future. Meanwhile, the great majority of renal-failure patients remain on hemodialysis machines, hooked to and dependent upon them either chronically or continuously, often at discouragingly great expense and inconvenience, even though dialysis is not desired by physicians or their patients, because of a lack of donors — both living and post mortem.

The first kidney transplants were called immoral or premature, as the Wright brothers were at Kitty Hawk. The same was said of Harvey Cushing's intercranial surgery, and of open-heart techniques in thoracic surgery. At the focal point of debate right now are heart transplants, evoking fear and reaction. The medical authority in the Soviet Union (Boris Petrovsky, Minister of Health), for example, once prohibited heart transplants until the rejection mechanism had been conquered. But in some of these failures of organ function, such as the heart's, to do nothing means odds of 100% against the patient, whereas to go ahead offers even at this stage a 40% chance of rescue in some cases (kidneys) and 20–40% in hearts. (There is some evidence that hearts are less vulnerable than kidneys to tissue rejection, but it is too early to be sure.) At a recent meeting on Significant Developments in Medicine and Surgery at the Boston Museum of Science, the physicians and surgeons and laymen there voted nine to one to persevere in their attempts to solve transplantation problems.

Organic transplants are by no means only experimental; by now they are therapeutic — for indeed, all treatment is a mixture of the two. We cannot escape the calculations of "statistical morality" or "mathematicated decisions" or "risk-gain" or "cost-effectiveness" choices, unless, of course, we are dealing with obvious and open-and-shut ethical questions which are entirely nonproblematic. How many such are there? (People who live by rules and principles think they can escape the problematic or, at least, the burden of facing it.) But in health and medical care there is no escape from diagnosis and prognosis. We can learn from the "book" but we can't *go* by it [see 15].

MORALS AND MEDICINE

No significantly different ethical questions are posed by other forms of spare-parts medicine such as endocrines, lungs and livers, or by non-organic transplants or grafts such as blood, blood vessels (arteries and veins), bones, cartilage, and corneas. Lung transplants have been tried seven times (twice in the United States, once in Canada, once in Edinburgh, and three times in Japan) but with no success as yet. On the other hand, a thymus from a thirteen-week-old girl was recently flown from London in a cold saline solution, and transplanted to a seven-month-old boy. Artery grafts are generally operational, as in the UCLA procedure by Dr. Kaufman and Dr. Moloney to bypass plugged kidney arteries with autotransplants or, sometimes, even with synthetic materials like dacron. A purely descriptive account of medical-surgical progress, especially with technology's help, would be fascinating but take too much space [see 12:132–150].

Even when there is no irrational objection to making a donation of tissue and organs, i.e., even though it is not looked upon as evil or undesirable in itself intrinsically, there are still occasional or situational moral questions involved extrinsically. Let us look now at four of these questions which can easily be raised even by those who are willing, everything else being equal, to contribute spare parts. They are: 1) the risks entailed, 2) the problem of competent consent, 3) the principles of selection, given the scarcity or low supply problem, and 4) the ethical status of xenografts from animals, or interspecific organs and tissue. (This fourth one is really a pseudo-ethical question, but it merits a brief mention. It is "pseudo-ethical" because it judges values not by their functional or effective nature (consequences), but by some assigned inherent or "intrinsic" feelings about their "nature" regardless of consequences. Thus: "It is just *wrong* to put something from a pig into a person; I just *know* it.")

As for the risks taken, they can be both psychological and physical. In *inter vivos* transplants of kidney, for example, the donor reduces his renal survival potential by half (but not his functional powers), and this might become a source of anxiety. If the donor is related to the recipient the motive might be guilt compulsion rather than true loving concern, and thus result in delayed reactions or too late regrets. A recipient or donor may unconsciously not want to "share spares" with the other, and end up with destructive hostility feelings.

The physical risks are not very great. Wives or husbands often object to their spouses' "cutting down their survival chances" for a third person's sake, fearful for themselves or their dependents. Actually, if the donor subsequently develops the same organic failure he can be "rescued" too, in his turn. And the risk in the operation is very slight. Suturing in dogs is more difficult than in humans, yet hundreds are sutured successfully to every human being. Replantation, as of a severed hand, is more exacting than organ transplantation, and open-heart surgery is more difficult than heart transplants. After all, the risk rate in everything is always finite, and cannot be reduced to zero; even in general anaesthesia it remains at 1:1,500. (There is even one instance on record of a recipient becoming pregnant with a zygote from a transplanted ovary!) Risks to donors can be cushioned by insurance underwritten by the public health authority, thus reducing the fears of physicians and hospitals as well. As Dr. George Reed of New York University once said of heart transplants, when sound criteria are applied and calculations of loss-gain made, do we have a "moral right" *not* to try a transplant, or to be a donor?

The risk, or more carefully phrased, the danger of rejection after transplantation, is always a part of the situation. The antigens are built genetically right into the cell nuclei. Blood typing, quite apart from the "throwing" problem, eliminates about 50% of prospective donors in a given case, with about 10% of available donors being compatible. This is a fact about transplantation which underlies the crucial importance of a wide choice of living or cadaveric donors being available. Only occasionally is a "well" kidney removed for purposes of treatment of non-renal ills, but these should be reported alertly by doctors, nurses, and hospital chaplains. Progress in immunosuppression has been steady. One interesting line of inquiry has been suggested by the fact that mothers usually do not reject the foetus for nine months even though it is alien tissue. (Some speculate that the key is to be found in the placenta.)

Consent is a common ethical consideration in all medicine, especially in surgery and clinical experimentation [see 9]. But it takes on an added dimension in matters of tissue donation. "Competent" consent legally and ethically is a matter of free choice (non-coercive and voluntary) and understanding of what is at stake ("informed"). Treatises on the subject follow an almost conventional pattern. For example, sometimes moralists decide that prisoners in penitentiaries are in the very nature of their situation not really free to be voluntary donors. Sometimes they say that patients are so influenced by physicians, even when the physician leans over backwards not to influence the patient, that they will make donations because "Doctor seems to want it" — not because they themselves do.

In almost any medical situation the patient will be able to understand only a part of what the facts and the probabilities are. Thus, competent consent should not be understood in an ideal or perfectionist way which makes it practically impossible. (There is far less reason to fear coercion or ignorance when the consent is for a future donation post mortem.) There will never be a fully "competent" consent given: while it should never be perfunctory it will always have to be substantial rather than perfect, on any model.

A DEADLY SCARCITY

This paper is concerned with a deadly scarcity of organs and living donors. That is not too strong a way to put it. At Peter Bent Brigham Hospital, according to Dr. Francis D. Moore, only two or three renal transplants can be done per month. The result is the institution (it has come to that, literally) of selection committees. They may be made up of and by hospital medical people, or more broadly if appointed by a public authority. (For example, there is one in the state of Washington, set up by the Governor to decide which kidney patients are to have access to a limited supply of dialysis machines and new kidneys.) Their task is to decide who shall live, and who shall die. The lack of donations often makes selection exactly that grim and portentous. Our ignorance or indifference saddles responsible people with just such a tragic burden.

The principles of selection to be followed are under debate. Shall machines or organs go to the sickest, or to the one with most promise of recovery; on a first come first served basis; to the most "valuable" patient (based on wealth, education, position, what?); to the ones with the most dependents; to women and children first; to those who can pay; to whom? Or should lots be cast, impersonally and uncritically? Can we get away from questions of counter-productivity and cost-effectiveness? If we don't think people ought to be making such dread decisions about other people, should we not be calling from the housetops for more donors?

Recently in Leeds, England, three aortic valves from a pig's heart were used in a 38-year-old mother's heart, quite successfully. One patient lived over nine and a half months on a chimpanzee's kidney [34]. An ape's heart valves were used in a 17-year-old young man in Budapest in 1968. A pig's liver was used in Johannesburg for a 47-year-old woman, but not transplanted; it was used outside her body, to perfuse her blood and at once it brought her out of coma. The tale of interspecific transplants could go on and on. Any objection to the practice must be based on irrational or a-rational sentiment; it is, indeed, only a pseudo-problem. For those who are thus prejudiced it is enough simply to point out that they had better be more vigorous in recruiting donors! More progress is being made in mechanical hemodialysis, for example, which is only a holding maneuver for patients, than in getting *people* to help people. We can build machines more easily than we can rally donors to help their fellow men. This is a *real* ethical problem. Who has a right to complain about xenografts, if he has not offered to help by sharing human parts?

Mention of artificial organ-function opens another area we cannot explore here as much as it deserves. News reports of heart transplants in the past year have familiarized Americans with such devices as the resuscitative heart-lung machine which can keep organs going viably after "death" has occurred — whether determined by a clinical or cerebral definition. After a donor's death his heart can go on a respirator, keeping respiration and circulation going for hours after the brain is gone. (This is the reason for a cerebral definition of death.) In the same way machines can contribute enormously to the solution of such problems as the storage and preservation of organs ("stockpiling")

— e.g., the freezing-perfusing machines developed at the University of Minnesota Medical Center.

Dr. Willem Kolff, a pioneer in devising successful dialysis machines, now asserts that by 1970 there will be artificial kidneys, inexpensive and so simple and convenient that patients themselves can put them together and operate them for chronic use. Dr. Denton Cooley of St. Luke's Hospital in the Texas Medical Center in Houston believes that the ultimate solution to failing hearts is the mechanical and implantable heart, even though transplants will remain routine for at least five years. There is nothing wild or visionary about these predictions, not just for the artificial kidney but others as well. Full scale work on artificial implanted hearts has progressed impressively under sponsorship of the National Institutes of Health. There is no artificial liver in view, but for most other organs the field is wide open.

DEATH AND TIME

The crucial question — how are we to understand death? — obviously has a bearing on the problem of an adequate supply of human tissue. A great deal of the fear that timid people have, that transplanters may redefine death in order to hasten the donor's death in terminal decline, results from the pressures due to the lack of organs — although the objectors rarely acknowledge what the obstruction is. Brain death, as recommended by many in modern times, calls for waiting twenty-four hours or so with a reconfirmed flat electroencephalograph reading [31]. But a cadaveric heart has to be used sooner than that, unless put on a machine. For kidneys, twenty-eight hours is the longest interim period between the donor's death and transplant thus far, before ischemia, the stoppage of blood flow and consequent anemia, ruins the tissue.

A Dominican father, Damien Boulogne, a seminary professor of philosophy, got a new heart at Hôpital Broussais-La Charité in Paris in 1968. In *La Vie Catholique,* as reported in the press, he wrote that the donor is not "sacrificed" as some say, "He has already been in a closed circuit [the heart-lung machine] for days, and is therefore already dead. . . . His survival is artificial. No problem" [40:50]. Boulogne called the heart "an admirable pump, but 'stupid,' a machine having its own circuit." The same could be said of all organs, except the brain.

Dr. Cooley, who has supervised more heart transplants than any other surgeon, and with a higher proportion of survival success than anybody else, put it this way: "The heart has always been a special organ. It has been considered the seat of the soul, the source of courage. But I look upon the heart only as a pump, a servant of the brain. Once the brain is gone, the heart becomes unemployed. Then we must find it other employment" [23:34]. At a grand rounds in March, 1968, I heard him say, "When the brain is gone there is no point in keeping anything else going."

This is, of course, the classical view of life or the soul (*psyche*) in the western doctrine of man, a rational view reflected in, for example, a great deal of Catholic philosophy. We can hark back to Byron's lines, "Maid of Athens, ere we part, give O give me back my heart," and a witty critic's remark that the Greeks thought the liver and not the heart was the seat of the "soul" or person. He therefore proposed a paraphrase of Byron, "Maid of Athens, ere we sever, give O give me back my liver." Now it is time for a second paraphrase, in the light of modern medicine: "Maid of Athens, ere we're twain, give O give me back my brain." It is the encephalograph, not the cardiograph, which tells us whether "anybody is there" or not.

Much of the pressure behind new proposals for a cerebral definition or "brain death" (irreversible coma) comes from the time factor. "Functional death" is a new concept emerging because resuscitative methods can keep hearts or livers or kidneys going in comatose patients after the brain has quit. This maintenance is necessary so that cadaveric transplant organs can remain in "health" until they are excised and transferred to the recipient patient. The dead donor is not alive in any meaningful sense, whether it is a case of artificially keeping the organ function going when it would otherwise cease or of restarting it after it has stopped.

Time is of the essence. Just getting an organ from one hospital to another is often touch-and-go. In most cases only a two or three hour interval after death is possible in kidney transplants, although there is a record of 28 hours for one kidney after excision, *in vitro*. Even cooled to 4° C–6° C a kidney's circulation must be restored in from 75 to 90 minutes. Making sure the donor is "dead" may ruin his organ as far as the recipient goes; hurrying it up may "murder" the donor by the old-fashioned clinical tests of death [see 19]. At the Karolinske Hospital in Stockholm in 1965 a kidney was removed for transplant and the doctor in charge was accused of "contributing" to the donor's death, and tried in court. A nationwide TV debate began: "Have we the right to remove vital organs from a dying person if by doing so we can save another person's life?" Physicians and ethicists generally said "Yes."

All will hang, of course, on what we mean by "a dying person" and it is high time we faced up to it. The conventional wisdom holds that we may not "hasten" a donor's death, but what. is it to "hasten" death when we have methods now that both suspend death and reanimate after it? And in any case, surely it is ethical to speed things up, once the donor is *in terminus*, if he has foreseen such a situation and consented not only to the transplant but to the speeding up.

> [Dr. Louis Lasagna says, "Legally, there is no way for the physician to hasten death, even if the patient requests it and the family approves of it" [22:224]. Here Lasagna refers to euthanasia, but it bears morally on not only one's freedom to end useless suffering but also on *one's obligation to save lives by giving useful tissue inter vivos*, for some procedures.]

(Some doctors might not "like" to do this and certainly ought not to be required to, *if they provide for their replacement*. And some lawyers will argue that it is against both common and statute law; the legal side still needs settling, since medical reality is so far ahead of legal concepts.)

Scarcity and speed. Each one is a problem that donors could and should alleviate. More people should be counseled to donate, and they should include as much freedom to act for lifesaving in their terms as possible. Every state has a statute of frauds which lists enforceable conditions of contract or promise, and what must be solemn (in writing) and the like. To quote Jean de la Bruyère, "Liberality consists less in giving a great deal than in gifts well timed."

Current law hampers medical progress in its restriction on the use of cadavers and organs. No socially arranged and supported way has been worked out to solicit, secure, and distribute bodies for transplant, therapy, research, and instruction. Yet Dr. William Likoff, a recent president of the American College of Cardiology, estimates that about 50,000 patients a year could benefit from new hearts.

The present jumble of state laws has incited a meeting (in Philadelphia, July, 1968) of medical and legal specialists to draft a "uniform anatomical gift act" which is to be put before the National Conference on Uniform State Laws and other legal bodies. Thirty-eight states have adopted general gift statutes to guarantee that the deceased's gift will not be denied by next of kin; four states have laws only for donating eyes; others have none. But they all vary in important respects. Next of kin have been the moral bottleneck in Anglo-American law ever since the temporal courts threw out the church's probate jurisdiction over bodies (a change that took place in the late eighteenth century). Such a uniform law as proposed would also help to protect physicians from next of kin trouble, since body taboo is still tragically persistent.

SOME COMFORT FOR BAD CONSCIENCE

Cadaveric transplants and artificial organs and tissue, rather than *inter vivos*, will bypass (not answer) most of the ethical questions. They eliminate the issue over "hastening death" — at least in most cases — and the doubts about reducing the donor's survival potential. They reduce the need to put "pressure" on patients to give organs, especially in preterminal stages. Early testamentary disposition takes care of the consent problems, understanding and freedom. It relieves next of kin from decision making. It entails no risk of disease or debility due to the transplantation. It obviates any legal suits in torts or claims. There is no cost to the donor in time, money, or conscience. It reduces guilt in family or friends unwilling or afraid to dispose of the donor's tissue. And so on.

But the big relief will come when human beings are no longer needed to help human beings, either by ante or post mortem help. The fact is that more progress is being made in devising artificial ways to save life than in getting human help with spare parts. But it is also true that there is greater promise of spare parts from animals than from humans. Just as herds of horses are specially raised for steaks on many luncheon tables (the Harvard faculty club's, for one), so herds of baboons and gibbons and cows and swine will be raised specially for tissue and organs transplantable into humans. Bio-engineers doing polymerization for chemically-constructed tissue and electronic engineers devising organ-substitutes, as well as dumb animals, can be counted on to help people caught in serious tissue loss and organic failure in ways human beings cannot be counted upon.

The use of interspecific material, however — and the use of human tissue too — will be greatly enhanced as the methods of preservation are worked out. It is not feasible yet to "bank" material for any length of time by freezing or hypothermia, since water in cell tissue expands on freezing and ruptures the membranes. Perhaps an antifreeze substance like glycerol will solve it. (In the Navy's center at Bethesda, Maryland, organs are being attached to baboons to keep them going until the recipient is ready. And polio vaccine is developed in monkey tissue now.)

Continuous storage by freezing or perfusion is not solved for whole organs, and it is possible only for a few weeks even with skin, sperm, and vessels. It is easier, of course, for bone, cartilage and corneas. Successful animal experiments were reported recently which show that human organs could be stored as long as

72 hours, and indefinite freezing may be about a decade away. Further, surgeons at the University of Minnesota in August, 1968, at a meeting of the Society for Cryobiology, exhibited machines about the size of an automatic washer which cool, pressurize, oxygenate, and supply blood to tissue and organs. These machines lengthen the time of preservation and expedite shipping interstate or cross-country [32]. It is *this* kind of thing which medicine is counting on, not human generosity.

Many of the states with anatomical and tissue gift acts have specific forms. These forms often provide for tests and procedures *before* death to make transplantation more effective, and a direction to "my Administrator, Executor, or next of kin to carry out this bequest" immediately upon death [see 36]. They are to be witnessed and signed in accordance with the rules of all such legal instruments. Copies are usually given to the family physician, a close friend or relative, and a hospital or medical college. In certificates bequeathing one's body to a medical school, some such provision as the following is often included:

> Should circumstances at the time of my death make desirable and practical the transplanting or preserving of any parts or tissue of my body to assist with the life and health of other human beings my physician is authorized to arrange this, subject, if time permits, to the approval of the Medical College whose needs he shall, in any event, keep actively in mind.

Dr. Marion Collins has issued over 200,000 bracelets or necklace tags from the Medical Alert Foundation in Turlock, California. These are devices to alert doctors in emergency services that a wearer is diabetic, hemophiliac, or allergic — as to penicillin. The tags or "uni-body cards" also say that the wearer will donate an organ or tissue (e.g., cornea), and the Foundation's telephone switchboard is open day and night to inform hospitals as to which organs are transplantable, blood types, and the like. In Sweden, Ingemar Hedenius, a philosopher, further proposes *dodshjalp* (death help) in the form of a notice that one wishes euthanasia or to be "let go" in terminal illness.

A rather bizarre offshoot of all this is the Life Extension Society. It publishes a newsletter, *Freeze-Wait-Reanimate.* Its founder, Robert Ettinger, professes to use cryogenics as a way to freeze the bodies of its members after death by liquid nitrogen, and then to "resurrect" them by artificial resuscitation when a cure has been found for whatever fatal malady struck them down. (Capsules to hold the bodies cost $4,000, plus $150 annually to maintain them.) One woman says, "With bad luck, I'll stay simply dead. With good luck, I may live again. It's worth trying" [39]. A half-dozen or more of those who have signed up have now been frozen in this long range lay-away plan in the Society's facilities in Phoenix and New York. It makes an interesting gamble, with heavy hazards on two counts: 1) finding the cure, and 2) reanimating the corpse. How the odds are set is undisclosed.

Their gamble is, of course, a new version of Pascal's Wager: "If I profess faith in God and eternal life and there is none, I lose nothing; if I profess this faith and it is grounded in fact, I gain everything; therefore I believe."

It is well known that funeral directors are opposed to bequests for dissection, and for obvious reasons. The "bier barons," as they have been called, are threatened by an ethical attitude to death, as distinguished from a religious one [see 41]. As one leading "mortician" has said, "With no body, there is no funeral. If there are no funerals, there are no funeral directors" [27:281]. On the other hand, Howard C. Rather, president of the National Funeral Directors' Association, says that it is quite possible to prepare bodies and have a regulation funeral after transplant. Nevertheless, embalmers complain. Not only transplants but autopsies remove veins and arteries and cranial separation in autopsies, and this greatly adds to the problems of the embalmer, who finds it easiest, of course, to inject his fluids in a single and undivided system. They do not, however, openly complain or quarrel when autopsies and donations occur, but they do put pressure on whenever they can do so without controversy. Funerals are a wholesale waste of human tissue, pagan and barbaric. The ideal of a rational and theologically disciplined ethics would be to eliminate funerals (burial or cremation), but a realistic standard our culture can and would allow, would be to give dissection and donation first claims, with funerals to adjust accordingly. This ought not to be too much more threatening than the growing appeal, notably unwelcome to the morticians and florists and their profit account, "Please omit flowers."

MAKING DECISIONS, PLAYING GOD

The troglodyte and "rear-view mirror" reaction to all this is, "You are playing God." Perhaps we should simply accept this description of what it means to use our new controls over life and death in a responsible way. The real question is *which* God we are playing when we shoulder the solemn and often perplexing burden of making vital decisions. It is "the God of the gaps," as theologians say, whose role and prerogatives we are preempting. This God is a hypothesis of ignorance, the honor we pay to what we do not know or cannot do, born and projected out of our feelings of awe and fear of the unknown — the *mysterium tremendum*. As we have learned and succeeded, that God has diminished and died. The God of the gaps is dead.

This is not a human or demonic pretension. On the contrary, the advance of our medical powers serves a humble and serious concern to be responsible, to respond to need effectively. Less and less do people die or suffer stupidly and helplessly, trapped in a value-blind "nature." Man's intelligence transcends nature progressively. And we might note that nothing is won by moderate counsel to "go slow" in our conquest of illness and death. The errors of moderate opinion are often harder to detect than those of extreme opinion, and for that reason they are often far worse and more dangerous, and certainly more likely to disarm us. ("Extreme" in this context usually means logical or rational or courageous.)

Every ill person, if free to choose life or a chance for it *in articulo mortis*, ought to be free likewise to choose *not* to go on living or to be brought back by resuscitation and transplant. On the other hand, he has less freedom or right, ethically, to refuse such a chance for others — for example, by giving his body or tissue. We might choose death for ourselves more rightly than we can choose it for others. This is exactly what a refusal or failure to be a donor, in one way or another, amounts to — choosing death for somebody else. Death is not always evil; it can sometimes be a friend [11]. But friends are chosen, not imposed. After all Montaigne was correct, "Death is but an end to dying." Or in Hester Piozzi's terms, "A physician can sometimes parry the scythe of death, but has no power over the sand in the hourglass" [33].

The Convocation of Canterbury, Church of England, has voted to provide "pastoral guidance to those who bequeath their bodies for research or who wish parts of them to be available for transplants, and to those who have to make funeral arrangements when such use is made of their bodies."

Edwin Diamond once said, "Change seems to come only when some determined health group publicizes its advantages and orchestrates consent" [7]. That orchestration, in a firm campaign waged against our shameful waste of human tissue, could be provided by ministers, chaplains, doctors (especially general practitioners), teachers, public health officials, publicists, and many others whose support of medicine and paramedical genius can still overcome the mini-morality of body taboo.

REFERENCES

1. Aiken, Henry D: *Reason and Conduct* (Alfred A Knopf, Inc, New York, New York) 1962.
2. Bonifazi, Conrad: *A Theology of Things* (Lippincott, Philadelphia, Pennsylvania) 1968.
3. I Corinthians 15:44.
4. Couch, N P: Supply and Demand in Kidney and Liver Transplantation, *Transplantation*, vol 4, no 5, Sept 1966, pp 587–595.
5. Cunningham, Fr B J: *Morality of Organic Transplantation* (Catholic University Press, Washington, D.C.) 1944.

6. Cyborg. From the Greek words meaning an instrument to govern or steer, or a functional control device.

7. Diamond, Edwin: Are We Ready to Leave Our Bodies to the Next Generation?, *The New York Times Magazine*, Apr 21, 1968.

8. Elkinton, J Russell: editorial, *Annals of Internal Medicine*, vol 60, no 2, pt 1, Feb 1964, p 309.

9. Fletcher, John: Human Experimentation Ethics in the Consent Situation, *Law and Contemporary Problems* (Duke University, Durham, North Carolina) vol 32, no 4, 1967, pp 620–649.

10. Fletcher, Joseph: Donor Nephrectomies and Moral Responsibility, *Journal of the American Medical Women's Association*, Nov 1968.

11. Fletcher, Joseph: Elective Death, in E Fuller Torrey, ed: *Ethical Issues in Modern Medicine* (Little, Brown & Co, Boston, Massachusetts) 1968, pp 139–157.

12. Fletcher, Joseph: Medicine's Scientific Developments and Ethical Problems, in Dale White, ed: *Dialogue in Medicine and Theology* (Abingdon Press, Nashville, Tennessee) 1968.

13. Fletcher, Joseph: *Moral Responsibility* (Westminster Press, Philadelphia, Pennsylvania) 1967.

14. Fletcher, Joseph: *Morals and Medicine* (Beacon Press, Boston, Massachusetts) 1961, esp chaps 5, 7.

15. Fletcher, Joseph, and Hofling, Charles K: Human Experiments — Some Questions of Ethics, *Postgraduate Medicine*, vol 43, no 3, Mar 1968, pp 80–85.

16. Freehof, Solomon B: *A Treasury of Responsa* (Jewish Publication Society of America, Philadelphia, Pennsylvania) 1962.

17. Healy, E J, SJ: *Medical Ethics* (Loyola University Press, Chicago, Illinois) 1956.

18. Jacobowitz, Immanuel: *Jewish Medical Ethics* (Philosophical Library, New York, New York) 1959. It is worth noting that in this comprehensive work there is nothing about the "lawfulness" of transplants. But the Jewish silence

does not always imply disapproval, and a good guess is that Reform Jews will eventually endorse it.

19. *Journal of the American Medical Association*, vol 204, no 6, May 6, 1968, p 539, editorial.
20. Kelly, Gerald, SJ: *Medico-Moral Problems* (Catholic Hospital Association, St Louis, Missouri) 1958.
21. Kelly, Gerald, SJ: Pius XII and the Principle of Totality, *Theological Studies*, vol 16, Sept 1955, pp 373–396, presents complications and difficulties in this "doctrine."
22. Lasagna, Louis: *Life, Death and the Doctor* (Alfred A Knopf, Inc, New York, New York) 1968.
23. *Life*, Aug 2, 1968.
24. Lynch, J J, SJ: Human Transplantation: A Theological Observation, *Linacre Quarterly*, vol 35, no 2, May 1968, pp 122–125.
25. McCarthy, John: The Morality of Organic Transplantation, *Irish Ecclesiastical Record*, vol 67, Mar 1946, pp 192–198.
26. McFadden, Charles J, OSA: *Medical Ethics* (Davis, Philadelphia, Pennsylvania) 1961.
27. Mitford, Jessica: *The American Way of Death* (Simon & Schuster, New York, New York) 1963.
28. Murray, J E, and Barnes, B A: Introductory Remarks on Kidney Transplantation, *Transplantation*, vol 5, no 4, 1967, p 824.
29. Murray, J E; Barnes, B A; and Atkinson, J: Fifth Report of the Human Kidney Transplant Registry, *Transplantation*, vol 5, no 4, pt 1, 1967, pp 752–754.
30. Murray, J E; Merrill, J P; and Harrison, J H: Renal Homotransplantation in Identical Twins, *Surgical Forum*, vol 6, 1954, p 432.
31. *The New York Times*, Aug 4, 1968.
32. *The New York Times*, Aug 6, 1968.
33. Piozzi, Hester Lynch Thrale: *A Letter to Fanny Burney*, Nov 12, 1781.
34. Reemstma, K, *et al*: Renal Heterotransplantation in Man, *Annals of Surgery*, vol 160, no 384, 1964.

35. Soloveitchik, Joseph B: The Lonely Man of Faith, *Tradition* (Rabbinical Council of America) vol 7, no 2, summer 1965, p 53n.

36. Stickel, Delford L: Ethical and Moral Aspects of Transplantation, *Monographs in the Surgical Sciences*, vol 3, no 4, 1966, pp 296–297, appendices D, E.

37. *Theologia Moralis*, II.

38. *Time*, Aug 27, 1965.

39. *Time*, Sept 30, 1966.

40. *Time*, July 26, 1968.

41. Warner, W Lloyd: *The Living and the Dead: A Study of the Symbolic Life of America* (Yale University Press, New Haven, Connecticut) 1959, esp pp 302 – 318, on the "transition technicians" — funeral directors, embalmers, doctors, ministers, and priests.

42. *Yearbook* (Central Conference of American Rabbis, New York, New York) 1953.

2. ON UPDATING DEATH

by Paul Ramsey

HELEN LANE DIED of cancer more than fifteen years ago. Yet she is living in the cellular meaning of life, and today she is still called by her proper name in laboratories all over the world. Cancer researchers use the logo "HeLa" for this line of cells, composed of the first two letters of the two names by which she was known and addressed when otherwise alive. This woman's cells live on, each having the genotype that constituted all her generic and individual attributes; in a sense she still has the cancer that once was said to have caused her death. It was Dr. George Guy of Johns Hopkins University who bestowed upon her this factitious "immortality" and, it may well be, the capacity for her life to be of unique service to humanity long after her "moment of death." Thus Helen Lane is probably the most ubiquitous human being in the world, at least since the Lutherans declared that the risen body of Christ possesses the attribute of omnipresence belonging to God the Father!

But cellular life is not what we mean by being alive. To pronounce someone dead never required waiting for cellular death finally to occur. Clinically, life means the functioning of the integrated being or physiological organism in some sense as a whole. Clinical death means the cessation of this functioning. This in turn depends on the functioning of certain great organ systems.

It was widely assumed, at least until the recent spate of suggestions for revising the meaning of clinical death, that spontaneous cardiac activity, spontaneous respiratory activity, and the spontaneous activity of the brain and central nervous system were the indications of life. The irreversible cessation of the functioning of heart and lungs and brain was required before anyone was pronounced dead. The death of other great organ systems, such as the liver or kidneys, caused the death of the individual through a fatal effect upon the essential functions of heart and lungs and brain. Generally speaking, these indications of the moment of death were themselves not sorted out, or one given priority over the others. Cardiovascular, respiratory, and brain activity are known to be interdependent, but they are not always coincident in cessation. Therefore, a physician checked all three in determining the presence of life or death. He did this by observing the movement of breathing in the patient or by a mirror to detect slight emissions of breath; by listening for the heartbeat or by electrocardiogram; and by testing for reflex action or by electroencephalograph. Then in the absence of these signs of life and the impossibility of reviving them, a patient would be declared to be dead.

These procedures may be significantly changed by the end of this decade. An increasing number of experts and committees of medical faculties or associations are calling for an updating of the meaning of death — or, if not for revision in the clinical concept of the "moment" or the "meaning" of death, for an updating of the clinical tests for determining that a patient has died.

The occasion for the unusual activity on this front is, of course, the fact that the use of human tissues in therapy and organ transplantation finally reached the heart. Dr. Denton A. Cooley, of St. Luke's Hospital, Houston, Texas, who himself directed the surgical team that has performed ten of the world's thirty-two heart transplants (as of August 20, 1968), expressed surprise that this medical achievement should have caused such a stir. The transplantation of the heart is only the culmination of (and this culmination doubtless itself a mid-point in) the use of human tissues in medical practice with its supporting medical research for the past four or five decades [see 8; 14]. It is an interesting question why the transplantation of the heart aroused so much more discussion, and indeed controversy, than was the case in regard to other vital organs.

The answer is deeper than sentiment. The site of love and the habitat of the soul — celebrated in the poetry and psalms of all ages — had now been replaced by a simple pump. What is man now that his heart has been reduced to a replaceable muscle? Lord Byron (high-tailing it out of Athens) could write: "Maid of Athens, ere we part,/ Give, O give me back my heart!/ Or, since that has left my breast,/ Keep it now and take the rest!" The heart seems an appropriate part to take for the whole, for the essential Byron. It would not have sounded the same if he had said, "Maid of Athens, ere we sever,/ Give, O give me back my liver!" Yet the liver is physiologically no less necessary than the heart for there to be life or any human being.

Not only in love poetry but in scripture and religious song the heart has human as well as physiological importance. This may lend a degree of support to the incipient feeling of a few of the surgeons that it was religious sentiment or mystique about the unknowable depths of sacredness in man, i.e., superstitious conceptions, that stimulated the public questioning of what was for them an ordinary cutting and suturing procedure and the next obvious step to be taken in patient care.

Yet it is perhaps with the primitive psycho-physiology of the Bible that we come close to understanding the problem of the meaning of life and death as it has arisen in modern medicine from the technique of organ transplantation. Deuteronomy 12:23 declares that "the blood is the life"; Leviticus 17:14 that "the life of all flesh is the blood thereof." Prophet and psalmist pray God to "try the reins," i.e., the kidneys, the site of conscience; the scriptures frequently speak of men's "bowels of compassion." And we are commanded to love the Lord our God with all our hearts, souls, minds, and strength. This primitive psychology distributing the capacities of man to the various organ systems was not only figuratively but literally meant; not only literally but figuratively. Everywhere it was *the life* that was at issue. The scriptures know no life that is not embodied; no man who in life is not (in Karl Barth's terms) the soul (the subject) of his body and the body of his soul. Neither does a contemporary physician know any other life in the practice of medicine and the care of his patients (whatever else he may say or think about the "soul"). Therefore I venture to say that Isaiah or Jeremiah would have understood the problem that arose for us dramatically in the late sixties of the twentieth century when tissue transplantation finally reached the heart.

It is life that has palpably been touched, and our understanding of life and death has been put in question. The astonishment as well as the concern that arose at once over the news of the first heart transplant is to be explained by the fact that the heart is an unpaired organ whose functioning is our life, and by the fact that it is an unpaired organ that "ticks." Because we feel its functioning, the heart has for us a significance that, for example, the liver (another unpaired and physiologically an equally indispensable organ) does not have. This is paralleled only by respiratory functioning, which gives the lungs a significance that similarly paired organs (e.g., the kidneys) do not have. Thus in human experience the "heart" and the "breath of life" have an importance that is attested to both by ancient lore and by the heart-lung machine. We feel both our breathing and our heartbeat; by comparison, we are only vaguely aware of the functioning of other great organ systems that may also constitute our being alive. It takes a greater sophistication to learn the central importance of the brain, for example, or to be persuaded to shift our concept of the meaning of life and death to brain life and brain death. This is what I mean by saying that because the heart is an unpaired organ that "ticks" it is understandable that grave human questions arose — questions of the meaning of life and death — when the heart was transplanted. Perhaps in principle these same questions were raised by open heart surgery, by the heart-lung machine, and by the insertion of artificial cardiac valves and tubes — in which procedures also the heart is stopped for hours and started again. It required the transplantation of the heart pump from one human being to another to heighten the imagination to apprehend what may be at issue in all these procedures; but what we apprehend by means of heightened imagination is the same thing, namely, the question whether heart function can or should be eliminated from the definition of being alive and being dead. This is the reason a number of proposals for updating the meaning of death have been stimulated by, or have found their "occasion" in, the transplantation of hearts.

DEFINITIONS AND TESTS

Proposals for updating death may be classified according to what they say about (1) the *meaning* of death and (2) the *criteria* for determining when death has occurred. It is one thing to propose a revision of the clinical *definition* of death and another to propose a revision of the *tests* for determining when a man has died. Some of the current proposals suggest the revision *both* of our understanding of physiological death and of the criteria to be used in pronouncing patients to be dead. Some suggest only that the tests be updated or refined.

Accordingly, it may be helpful to organize the current discussion under three main headings. The first position is the most radical, suggesting that the meaning of death be now understood as brain death and also that the criteria for determining this be shifted exclusively or almost exclusively to the electroencephalograph. This seems to be the view of a number of physicians, but it has not been endorsed, so far as I know, by any responsible committee appointed to study this question.

This most radical updating is commonly believed, however, to be more widely held than it actually is, because this point of view is incorrectly identified in the press with a second position. The latter would take the meaning of death to be brain death, but holds that there are a number of tests of irreversible brain death in addition to a patient's electroencephalogram taken at designated intervals of time.

Finally, it may be affirmed that the meaning of death is about what it always was, namely, the permanent cessation of heart, lung, and brain activity, but that the tests for determining death in this sense ought to be extensively refined and qualified for the protection of patients and physicians alike.

Before discussing the issues raised for medical ethics, it will be helpful to bring into view examples of these three positions.

1. According to a United Press International dispatch [9], a prominent neurosurgeon, Dr. James L. Poppen of the Lahey Clinic and New England Deaconess Hospital in Boston, who at the request of the White House, Vice President Humphrey, and Pierre Salinger flew to Los Angeles as a consultant concerning the late Senator Robert F. Kennedy's condition, said that it was his opinion that Senator Kennedy was legally and medically dead at 6:30 p.m. on Wednesday, June 5, 1968, eighteen hours after the shooting, but seven hours before he was officially declared dead at 1:44 a.m. on Thursday, June 6. It is true that at this news conference Dr. Poppen spoke of a number of other tragically important matters besides his reasons for this medical judgment, and his language may not at every point have made clear exactly what he meant. He said (if this news dispatch was correct) that when he first saw Senator Kennedy at 10 a.m. on Wednesday he "immediately" knew that he would not survive. On the other hand, he said that if the Senator had survived, his "intellectual faculties would not have survived," his bodily faculties would have been permanently impaired, and "he would have led a very grave and devastating existence." At the same time, Dr. Poppen offered it as his opinion that the Senator was a "dead man" from the moment he was hit, although the "destruction was not complete from the moment of impact."

However, to say that a man is irreversibly dying from destruction that has been set in course is not the same as making a present judgment that he is now irreversibly dead. Our attention should focus, therefore, on what according to Dr. Poppen happened at 6:30 p.m. on Wednesday to support the judgment that from that point on the Senator was "medically dead."

[I struck the word "legally" from the words of the news dispatch, since it is doubtful that the legal definition of death has so far been updated to support a verdict that a man is dead who still has a heartbeat, even if this be a reasonable medical proposal. A medical judgment that a man is dead is, of course, a legal judgment in the sense that the law itself acknowledges that only physicians can so declare. The law generally will and should support competent medical opinion in this matter; still, the law's endorsement of any revision of the meaning of death is necessary in determining legal death. This endorsement need not be by legislation; it can be by case law, or even by the law's silence in the face of changing medical practice.]

We should focus attention on the Senator's reported condition from this point on for seven hours until he was officially declared to be dead. Dr. Poppen said, as reported, that Senator Kennedy's electrical brain waves stopped at 6:30 p.m. on Wednesday and never started again, although his heart still beat.

In other words, although the heartbeat may have been faint and erratic, and although measures supportive of heart function may have been used in the effort to save him, it is not affirmed that there was an entire and an irreversible cessation of heart function at that time. This, then, is a neurosurgical redefinition both of the meaning of death and of the tests for this. Death means brain death, and the criteria for this are exclusively or almost exclusively brain tests. As reported, Dr. Poppen said that Senator Kennedy was legally and medically dead when the brain waves ceased (although his heart still beat).

In order to put to ourselves the question whether it would be right to update the definition of death to brain death alone and at the same time to narrow the criteria to brain tests alone, we have only to ask ourselves whether we would be willing to bury a man whose heart still beats [see 5:190]. Alternatively, we might ask whether we would be willing under similar conditions to remove one of man's vital organs for use as a "spare part" for another patient [see 2:69; 15:70]. The presence or absence of cardiac activity and other indices ought not hastily to be removed from our tests of whether a man is still alive or has died, even if our definition of death should be largely shifted to brain death. As David Daube has written, "The question of at what moment it is in order to discontinue extraordinary — or even ordinary — measures to keep a person alive should not be confused with the question at what moment a man is dead" or with the question of the meaning of the tests for death. "Discontinuation of such measures is often justifiable even while the patient is conscious" [5:190–191]. A decision to continue or to discontinue life sustaining treatment of a person who has suffered massive brain injury, or longer to sustain a comatose patient, is precisely a judgment made in the face of a life still present. It would be far more reasonable to open decisively the question under what conditions and by what means we should continue "heroic" efforts to save life than to construct an intellectual tour de force to pronounce a man dead whose heart still beats.

The proposed extensive updating of the definition of and the tests for death should also be contrasted with the manner in which a kidney was saved and used in a transplant operation from one David Potter, who suffered extensive brain damage in a brawl in June, 1963, at Newcastle upon Tyne [see 3; 6]. About 14 hours after admission on June 16 to the Newcastle General Hospital, Mr. Potter stopped breathing. "Artificial respiration was then begun by machine so that one of his kidneys could later be taken for transplantation in another man." I suppose this means that if he had not been placed on a respirator, he might at that point have been pronounced dead because of the cessation of spontaneous respiratory, cardiac, and brain function. On this supposition, there can be no decisive moral objection to the fact that "after 24 hours of artificial respiration a kidney was taken from the body on June 17. The respirator was then turned off. . . ."

Such a case may present only interim problems, because of the likely advancement in transplant technology. Still it is worth pondering. The German Lutheran theologian who has written most on medical-ethical questions, Helmut Thielicke, was commenting upon such a vital use of the body as a temporary "tissue bank" when he wrote:

It appears to me that one should not speak here of "maintaining alive." For we are concerned here with the maintenance of partial biological functions, or, to say it more pointedly, with the vital conservation of single organs of an unburied corpse. . . . One would say that in distinction to these partial "relics of life," the organism as a whole has ceased to be. And I now ask myself whether the means of such a vital conservation are fundamentally different from other forms of such conservation

— for instance, those employed in an institute of anatomy which are used for classroom purposes — are these fundamentally different from the vital quality [use] just indicated? This special method of conservation would then have to be understood as an achievement of modern medicine which knows how to maintain an organ within an irreversible and lethal over-all situation and is able again to make it productive by means of transplantation. It is beyond me why this should imply ethical or religious problems. The consciously chosen term "vital-conservation of individual organs" indicates, and is intended to indicate, that we are here concerned neither with anthropology nor with theology but rather with a question of biology which is dissociated from human values [17].

[An objection can be raised against this statement only because Thielicke (at ellipsis above) says, "Disregarding altogether any physiological definition of death. . . ."; and because his words "an irreversible and lethal over-all situation" are ambiguous as to whether he means to say that the man was irreversibly dying but was maintained alive for a time, or that the man was irretrievably dead but his organs were maintained alive for a time. It seems clear, however, that Thielicke really means to say that this is a case of "the vital conservation of the single organs of an unburied corpse." That *entails* a definition of physiological death.]

The difficulty in the Newcastle General Hospital case was that the coroner and the doctors were uncertain about what had happened or what was done to Mr. Potter; this, in turn, very clearly shows why the question of the meaning of death has been raised — occasioned — by organ transplants. The coroner was reported to have said that he thought Mr. Potter was alive when the kidney was removed on June 17, although there was no hope for him, but in his view, astonishingly, the doctors had committed no offense. The chief doctor, on the other hand, offered (it was reported) two views: (1) that Mr. Potter was "virtually dead" on June 16 when he ceased breathing, while he "legally" died when the heart ceased beating and the circulation ceased to flow on June 17 (when after the kidney had been taken the respirator was cut off), and (2) that he was "medically dead" on June 16 and "legally dead" on June 17. The legal correspondent of the *British Medical Journal* was principally concerned that these comments had opened up a difference between the legal and the medical definitions of death.

To the lay reader of this report it is, indeed, difficult to tell what happened or what was done to Mr. Potter. Because it is best to think the best of everyone, I can only suppose that on June 16 Mr. Potter, already lethally brain damaged, ceased to have spontaneous cardiac and respiratory functions. If so, then what followed was a case of (in Thielicke's words) "the vital preservation of single organs in an unburied corpse."

On July 24, 1968, the *Washington Post* reported concerning the transplant of the heart of a Houston housewife, Evelyn G. Krikorian, into the body of Fredi C. Everman of Arlington, Virginia, that Mrs. Krikorian had been dead for *four days* but that *her heart* was maintained alive during this period of time. In this case, the doctors thought they knew what they were doing. Mrs. Krikorian was dead because there was no natural heartbeat, no spontaneous breathing, no reflexes, and no brain waves (this is the third position on the meaning of death to be considered below). The respirator they used did not make a person live; it only kept *the heart* beating and the chest and lungs moving to supply oxygen to the blood. In short, the respirator was a means of sustaining a single organ in an unburied corpse. I shall argue in the sequel that the pronouncement of Mrs. Krikorian's death *or determining the criteria in terms of which such a judgment is to be made* should in no measure have had Mr. Everman's need in view. His need, however, can with proper precaution be made adjunct to what can properly be done with an unburied corpse.

It would, in truth, be an astonishing fruit of our technological civilization if *in mente* respirators and heart-lung machines became so integral a part of the "man alive" in his terminal illness that we could say that he "died" only when these machines were cut off, or (his brain by all indications damaged beyond recall) could say only that he was "virtually" dead when he irrevocably ceased to be capable of spontaneous cardiac-pulmonary functioning. These cases in any event are entirely different from the case of a man with extensive brain damage whose heart still beats from an entirely natural source. There is no need to resort to such an extensive updating of the meaning of death, especially not if we are capable of recalling other, more reasonable medical-ethical categories such as only caring for the dying to deal fittingly with untreatable terminally ill patients.

I shall argue in the sequel that there is sufficient need and sufficient reason in the dying or dead patient's own care, and that of his family, for clarifying or revising our understanding of death. The needs of potential recipients of organs need not and should not be brought into view even as adjunct considerations. Indeed, I am in this essay refraining from bringing the problems of transplantation under direct scrutiny and from making any final judgment about the ethics of giving and receiving, not taking, organs for transplants. We are concerned here with the problems of defining death, and the ethical issues that are raised.

2. On August 5, 1968, the *Journal of the American Medical Association* published a report of a committee of the Harvard Medical School, under the chairmanship of Dr. Henry K. Beecher, examining the definition of brain death. This article, entitled "A Definition of Irreversible Coma," expresses the view that death should be understood in terms of "a *permanently* nonfunctioning brain," but that there are many other — not only brain tests — for this [1]. A front page story in *The New York Times* announced that this special Harvard faculty committee recommended that the definition of death be based on " 'brain death,' even though the heart may continue to beat" [10]. The newspaper, in its summary of the news of the week the following Sunday, corrected this by saying that "in effect, the panel said that 'a permanently nonfunctioning brain' was tantamount to death, even though the heart and other organs may continue to function by *artificial means*" [12; italics added]. There is a world of difference between these two statements!

This illustrates the confusion that is widespread in the public

41

mind. It also brings us to the heart of the matter, the question of whether we should characterize a heart that still beats only because respiration is artificially maintained as a "spontaneously" beating heart (and so a sign of life) or by one step removed an "artificially" beating heart (and so *not* a sign of life, unless there is on this and other counts hope of restoring this and the other vital functions).

[In the *Daedalus* volume on "Ethical Aspects of Experimentation with Human Subjects," Dr. Beecher affirms that the crucial point was the Harvard committee's agreement that "brain death is death indeed, even though the heart continues to beat." Then the problem was for the committee to agree upon "the characteristics of a *permanently* non-functioning brain." In refining the tests for this, only *some* — perhaps a minority — of indefinitely comatose patients are rendered eligible to be declared dead. At the same time, and pertinent to these patients alone, Dr. Beecher affirms (among other characteristics) that "there are no spontaneous muscular movements or spontaneous respiration; *artificial respiration supports the continued heartbeat*" (*Henry K. Beecher,* "Scarce Resources and Medical Advancement," *Daedalus,* Spring, 1969, pp. 291, 293, italics added). Such a heart would seem to be more than "virtually" dead already. Some other committee, or Dr. Beecher himself, may want later to propose in the medical and the public forum valid ways to declare dead the other comatose patients who slip through the sieve of this committee's test for "no discernible central nervous system activity." Until this is done and further procedures for stating death agreed to, it seems that deeply comatose patients, the tragic "vegetable" cases whose respiration and hearts continue naturally, fall under an ethics of caring for the dying, the not yet dead, perhaps even the not yet dying. Then it would seem less confusing to say of the limited sort of cases dealt with by the Harvard report that they have no longer any capacity on their own to respirate, nor is there any hope of recovering either heart life or lung life. This, of course, is *because* their brains suffered such massive destruction.]

Defining death to mean, theoretically, the "permanent non-functioning of the brain" or a comatose condition in which there is "no discernible central nervous system activity," the committee then set itself the task of determining the "characteristics" of this state of affairs. It came up with a number of indications of this, and carefully laid out the procedures by which death, in the sense explained, could be determined in a combination of ways. It suggested three sorts or groups of "clinical signs" or criteria for brain death, and these are followed, only in the fourth place, by the electroencephalograph, which it should be noted "provides confirmatory data." A flat or isoelectric electroencephalogram is, of course, "of great confirmatory value" if expertly monitored, but an electroencephalograph is not always available. If available it is not enough. A complete "absense of cerebral function has also to be determined by purely clinical signs, to be described, or by absence of circulation as judged by standstill of blood in the retinal vessels, or by absence of cardiac activity."

In thus introducing its organization of the clinical tests of brain death, it seems very clear that the committee did not mean to exclude spontaneous circulation and spontaneous cardiac activity from among them. One can, it seems, shift the *meaning* of death entirely to the concept of a permanently nonfunctioning brain while still holding that the natural functioning of the other great organ systems are among the criteria for determining life or death in this sense. This the Harvard report says in effect when, in the summary, it states that "among the brain-stem-spinal mechanisms [i.e., still "discernible central nervous system activity"] which are conserved for a time, the vasomotor reflexes are the most persistent, and they are responsible in part for the paradoxical state of retained cardiovascular function, which is to some extent independent of nervous control, in the face of widespread disorder of cerebrum, brain stem, and spinal cord."

In addition to these expressed references to cardiovascular functioning as among the criteria determining whether a comatose individual has any discernible central nervous system activity, the committee's description of four "clinical signs" of brain death can hardly be verified in a patient whose heart still beats. These are: (1) No receptivity or responsivity, complete lack of response to the most intensely painful external stimuli and complete lack of any manifestation of "inner need." (2) No movement or breathing. Here we can see the meaning of "inner need": the total absence of spontaneous respiration in a patient on a mechanical respirator is established if, when the respirator is turned off for three minutes, there is "no effort" on the part of the patient to breathe spontaneously. Presumably the slightest effort to breathe (not success in doing so) would be taken as evidence of brain life, and *assisted* (as distinct from *artificial*) respiration would be resumed. (3) No reflexes. (4) Flat electroencephalogram. These clinical signs of brain life or death, and how properly to apply them, are described in great detail. Finally, it is suggested that all of the tests should be repeated at least twenty-four hours later with no change before a patient is declared dead.

As applied to the Newcastle General Hospital case, the Harvard report would quite properly require more than a determination that after the kidney was taken from Mr. Potter "the respirator was then turned off and there was no spontaneous breathing or circulation" [3]. It would require (1) three minute cut-offs to determine a failure of natural cardio-pulmonary function, repeated with no change at least twenty-four hours later, and (2) a declaration of death upon these evidences. *Then* the respirator could finally be turned off (or organs used in transplantation). The Harvard committee further suggests that "the decision to declare the person dead, and then to turn off the respirator, be made by physicians not involved in any later effort to transplant organs or tissue from the deceased individual."

Dr. Beecher has assured me that these tests can be verified in the presence of a "spontaneously" beating heart. That seems strange language to a layman. Still I am assured that there is plenty of clinical evidence that a man could "flunk" all the foregoing tests (and be declared dead) while his heart beats "naturally." This drives us to the crux of the matter, the question of the *term* we should use to best convey what the situation is. It is the respiration, artificial or natural, which alone prolongs the functioning of the heart. If the artificial respiration is prolonged beyond the point of no return of spontaneous respiration, how can the prolonged functioning of the heart be called spontaneous or natural or a permanent capacity of the patient?

I seriously suggest that subtly a radical change has taken place in the meaning of natural heartbeat as a test of life, and that this no longer means what it once meant, or still means in the case of patients not on respirators. It is the respirator that, one step away, is being rebutted by these tests, and not brain tests elevated or really spontaneous heart life downgraded in the procedures by which we should tell that a man has died. It is true that the respirator may be finally cut off in some sense "while the heart still beats"; but it is also cut off "while the lungs still breathe." The situation seems not unlike a "primitive case" of chest artificial respiration in which a scoutmaster abandons his efforts while a deeply brain-injured boy still has heart circulation, also while he still "breathes." But there is in either case no recoverable permanent capacity for either function.

The committee's recommendation seems to me to become confused only in a few passages in which artificially sustained heartbeat is taken to be a sign of life still in need of rebuttal. In past times, the report says, "the obvious criterion of no heart beat as synonymous with death was sufficiently accurate"; but "this is no longer valid when modern resuscitative and supportive measures are used. These improved activities can now restore 'life' as judged by the ancient standards of persistent respiration and continuing heart beat." These statements led to the misleading press interpretations of these recommendations. The "ancient standards of persistent respiration and continuing heart beat" meant natural or spontaneous heartbeat. The committee is not proposing that these be set aside. It is rather proposing careful checks upon whether these signs of life are or are not being restored by the use of modern resuscitative measures. It proposes that breathing and heartbeat entirely sustained by artificial means not be viewed as signs of life, and that a way be found to declare a person dead and these measures withheld.

We noted that Thielicke said that it is "beyond me" why the vital conservation of single organs of an unburied corpse should be thought to mean maintaining a man alive, or to involve the moral issues of life and death. In the same vein, I might remark that it is beyond me why an entirely artificial sustenance of breathing (and consequently of heartbeat) in an unburied corpse should be believed to be maintaining its "life" even to the extent the Harvard committee allows by using that word in quotation marks. This report is rather an eminently wise proposal for determining, in the face of these resuscitative measures, that the patient has died and that one is now only in the presence of an unburied corpse.

It was, therefore, also misleading for the committee to invoke the teachings of Pius XII on the dispensability of "extraordinary" means to save life, or for it to conclude (correctly, of course) that "it is the church's view that a time comes when resuscitative efforts should stop and death be unopposed." No longer to oppose death is not the same as first declaring a patient to be dead. There may be reasons under both heads for withholding "life" sustaining measures. This report's concern is to redefine death as brain death and to fix a plurality of tests for this, so that it can be judged that it is no longer *a life* that is being maintained, but only a corpse or only single organs (if transplant is in view).

[The news account of an interview with Dr. Henry K. Beecher on the day this report was published in the *Journal of the American Medical Association* stressed the connection of the proposed updating of death with the use of organs in transplants more than does the report itself [10]. I would argue that there is sufficient need and sufficient reason for (1) rethinking our understanding of death and/or (2) no longer opposing death, to be found in proper attention to the patient himself. There is no need — and in fact it is a little unsavory and may finally prove dangerous — to put behind these questions an urgency to answer them anew drawn in any measure from the question: "Can *society* afford to discard the organs of such patients if they can be used to restore health to salvageable patients" [13]?]

3. There is a third sort of possibility in redefining death. The concept or meaning of death itself may not be radically shifted

to brain death and at the same time the criteria for determining when a person has died may be held to be roughly what they always were (e.g., the cessation of the functioning of brain and heart and lungs), while it is argued that the several tests for declaring death to have occurred need to be greatly refined and *quantified* so that physicians can make this fateful decision with mathematical assurance. An illustration of this position can be found in the paper delivered at the convention of the American Medical Association in San Francisco, June 16, 1968, by Dr. Vincent J. Collins, director of the Division of Anesthesiology, Cook County Hospital, and Professor of Anesthesia, Northwestern University School of Medicine, entitled "Limits of Medical Responsibility in the Prolongation of Life: A Guide to Decision — A Dying Score" [7; 4].

[It is worth noting again the implication of the title of this paper, that the only limits upon medical responsibility in the prolongation of life are to be found in updating death — in this case producing "a dying score" to go by. There are sooner limits upon justifiable medical prolongation of life to be found in the dispensability of extraordinary means, as Professor David Daube pointed out. It is remarkable that extreme resuscitative and "life" sustaining measures should have become such a part of the patient's "life" that all the impulse toward the reform of medical practice goes into updating death (so that these measures can certainly be stopped), and there is little impulse to explore at the same time the medical-ethical categories governing when death should be unopposed and life prolonged no longer.]

Dr. Collins affirms that, if a patient is in deep unconsciousness related to severe illness or injury and if this is coupled with the diagnostic aspect of hopelessness on the physician's part, nevertheless "resuscitative techniques" and attempted reanimation procedures "must always be instituted as an immediate measure." The purpose of this is to "gain time" — for the patient, time for "the natural processes of restoration to work," and for the physician, "the time *for* decision and a time *of* decision." I should add also that treatment is a part of diagnosis, even under the aspect of hopelessness; proper diagnosis is a continuum of time acts accompanying attempted resuscitation. (If this is true no updating of our understanding of death, however radical, is going to cover or avoid every one of the tragic individual cases of patients successfully resuscitated to only a "vegetable" existence, or tell us what then to do. These cases call for reflection upon the possible justifications for withdrawing "heroic" treatment and allowing a patient to die. No redefinition of the meaning of death or of the criteria for judging that a man has died is going to remove the need for a doctor to include this most difficult thing as a part of his vocation: the conclusion that, in caring for the dying, death should not always be opposed.)

In his address, Dr. Collins defined clinical death as "the cessation of *integrated* life functions." He did not define death in terms of one or even several organ systems taken alone. This fitted in with the fact that the first stage in the dying process is simply a functional disorder or disequilibration of one or more organ systems in relation to the others. This disintegrated function has its onset before any intrinsic deterioration of an organ itself begins to take place. Then, says Dr. Collins, each organ has its own "vulnerability index" and "revival" time in the face of disequilibration in its interdependent functioning in relation to the other organs. The brain has a high degree of vulnerability to lack of oxygen and/or nutrition; the heart is the next most vulnerable organ.

With this understanding of the life or death of the organism as a whole goes the premise that "no single sign or function can or should be used to assess the capacity to live nor establish the state of death." Yet the capacity to live must be assessed and the state of death must be established. This leads to the proposal of "a dying score" based on five physiologic functions. These are listed "to some degree" in "an increasing order of dependance of one function upon the other": cerebral, reflex, respiratory, circulatory, and cardiac. Death means the cessation of these integrated and (in that order) dependent life functions. Each has to be assessed and is assigned a score for presence (2), potential (1) and absence (0). The complete and permanent absence (if it alone could be detected) of one of these functions would preclude the ability of the others to perform spontaneously. Despite this assertion, Dr. Collins proposes that only a o score for all five functions be regarded as "conclusive death." A score of 5 (i.e., 1 for each of the five functions, or if one is o, 2 for another of the functions), or more, represents potential life; while a score under 5 represents "impending" or "presumptive" death.

Finally, Dr. Collins recommends that these five functions be assessed at 15 minute intervals for up to two hours. An increasing score over a period of 1 to 2 hours indicates that the therapy is effective and the patient recovering, a decreasing score indicates failing therapy and the patient's deterioration, while, as we have said, o means conclusive death. Since the latter judgment seems conclusive enough, the importance of this "dying score" is to be found in (1) its reliance upon one or two hours of resuscitative measures to be sufficient to determine that a man has died, (2) its understanding of life and death in terms of the integrated functioning of the whole bodily being, (3) its employment of five physiologic criteria for determining the presence of life or death, and (4) the quantification of the assessments to be made. The last point seems to me to be a deceptive exactitude, since the numerical values simply indicate the "presence" or "absence" or "potential" ("depressed," "diminished," "abnormal," and "evoked response" are other terms used for score 1) for one of the five life functions. That was always the way a physician made the decision that a man had died, or waited to see.

A MORAL WARNING

In conclusion, I shall raise one simple ethical warning concerning these discussions of the meaning of death.

We have seen that the Harvard committee strongly recommends that "the decision to declare the person dead, and then to turn off the respirator, be made by physicians not involved in any later effort to transplant organs or tissue from the deceased individuals." This seems to be the unanimous opinion of all who have written or spoken on this subject. Will the care of a dying prospective donor tend to be any different because he *is* a prospective donor? This possibility, however remote, needs to be excluded altogether. The procedure to insure that a prospective donor's death be not *for this purpose* hastened is to establish a complete separation of authority and responsibility between the physician or group of physicians who are responsible for the care of the recipient and the physician or group of physicians who are responsible for the care of the patient who is a prospective donor. This is generally the procedure at medical centers where the organs of unburied corpses are used in transplantation. This safeguard was the principal point adopted at a recent meeting of the world Medical Assembly in Sydney, Australia, where there seemed from the press report to be lively discussion but little agreement on the meaning of death [11]. In other words, this procedure for insuring the protection of prospective donors is being recognized and adopted within the medical profession itself. It seems likely to be incorporated in legislation. The National Conference of Commissioners on Uniform State Laws is currently engaged in drafting a Uniform Anatomical Gift Act which, when approved in final form, probably in 1968, will include this principle of the "separation of powers" among its provisions [16:611]. It is hoped that this model bill will be adopted by the various state jurisdictions.

A comment from the point of view of religious ethics can only welcome this development. It is needed among the "checks and balances" in medical institutions in order to restrain and remedy wrongdoing. The fact that this was first widely recognized among the self-restraints physicians propose to place upon themselves, and which they affirm should in one way or another be imposed upon medical practice, shows that physicians are not on the whole believers in "participatory democracy" or in the aptness of human nature always to do the right without constraints that wisely and humanely impel them to do so.

But if this is so, what are we to say concerning updating the meaning of death, or the tests for determining when a man has died, today when great advancement is being made in organ transplantation? This is a development in the intellectual order, having important practical consequences for pronouncements of death. If in the practical order we need to separate between the physician who is responsible for the care of a prospective donor and the physician who is responsible for a prospective recipient, do we not need in the intellectual order to keep the question of the definition of death equally discrete from the use of organs in transplantation? If only the physician responsible for a dying man should make the determination that he has died, with no "help" from the medical team that has in its care a man who needs a borrowed organ, should not also the definition of death and the tests for it be ones that he thinks are sound or were agreed to by the profession without having transplantation in view? There would be too little protection of life attained in the practical order by entirely separating the authority and responsibility of the teams of physicians if the definition of death and the tests for it had already been significantly invaded by the requirements of transplant therapy. If no person's death should *for this purpose* be hastened, then the definition of death should not *for this purpose* be updated.

This is an ethical consideration of considerable importance. There is something not a little sinister when the press can state in explaining the Harvard report that the issue of the meaning of death has been "simmering" for some time but has presumably been brought to a boil by transplant therapy; that "many medical men fear that controversy will bedevil heart transplant efforts until the definition of death is clarified"; and quote Dr. Campbell Moses, medical director of the American Heart Association, to the effect that "until recently this was not critical, but we've got a whole new ball game now because two hours can make the difference in whether an organ is viable for transplant" [12]. If a person's particular moment of dying ought not to be run into that ball game (but ought rather to be separated from it by his own physician's independence of judgment), neither should the definition of death and of the tests for saying that a person has died. This ought to be a judgment and an agreement in medical science and practice that is also independent of whether organ transplantation is bedevilled, impeded or assisted thereby.

I was recently invited by a state medical association to submit in writing a theologian's definition of "the moment of death" to a symposium on that subject to be held in 1968. My reply, of course, was to say that a theologian or moralist as such knows nothing about such questions; that the determination of death is a medical matter; and that a theologian or moralist can only offer his reflections upon the meaning of respect for life, care of the dying, and some warnings of the moral complexities such as are set down here. The wording of this request seemed to me to be exceedingly significant. It said: "The purpose of this symposium is to more clearly define 'The Moment of Death' *so that* those sick people who need transplanted tissues will not be sacrificed because of a lack of a clear definition as to when the donor has died" [italics added]. This comes perilously close to unsavory talk about whether "*society* can afford to discard the organs of such [comatose] patients if they can be used to restore health to salvageable patients" [10].

This is not to say that the meaning of death need not be updated, or that the medical criteria for death do not need to be clarified. It is only to say that death should not be updated *for that purpose*. I should have thought that the purpose of a symposium to more clearly define the moment of death would be *so that* persons who have died need not have "life" sustaining measures inflicted upon their unburied corpses, needlessly and at great expense to their families. The reasons for this must be sufficient in themselves as proper medical practice. Any benefit that may accrue to other patients in this age of organ transplantation must be a wholly independent by-product of an updating of death that is already per se right and wise and a proper judgment to be made concerning the primary patient. The issues that have been "simmering" for a long time must be resolved as if transplantation did not exist as a surgical therapy. There is sufficient need and sufficient reason for updating death so that the primary patient and his family may be treated properly. There is sufficient need and sufficient reason, I have also suggested, for withholding (in the face of life and without a pronouncement of death) extraordinary measures in caring for the irreversibly dying.

Unless in the current discussion of the meaning of death the medical profession keeps these considerations clear of one another, it is apt to be convicted of an overweening desire to pass from one spectacular to another — from spectacular treatment of the dying, and indeed of the dead, to spectacular use of borrowed organs. It is apt to be convicted of failure to face the urgent problem of updating the meaning of death so long as it might have placed limits upon the use of extraordinary "life" sustaining measures, and then of radically revising the meaning of death and the tests for it when this would open the way to the use of other extraordinary life sustaining procedures for the sake of recipients, medical progress, and "society." If good must not only be done but also seem to be done, it can seriously be suggested that every prospect of organ donation be removed from discussion of any proposed needed revision in our understanding of death. That question can and should be allowed to rest on its own bottom.

REFERENCES

1. *Ad Hoc* Committee of the Harvard Medical School: A Definition of Irreversible Coma, *Journal of the American Medical Association*, vol 205, no 6, Aug 5, 1968, pp 85–88.
2. Alexandre, G P J: discussion of J E Murray: Organ Transplantation: The Practical Possibilities, in G E W Wolstenholme and Maeve O'Connor, eds: *Ethics in Medical Progress: With Special Reference to Transplantation*, Ciba Foundation Symposium (Little, Brown & Co, Boston, Massachusetts) 1966.
3. *British Medical Journal*, vol 2, Aug 10, 1963, p 394.
4. Collins, Vincent J: Limits of Medical Responsibility in the Prolongation of Life: A Guide to Decision — A Dying Score, *Journal of the American Medical Association*, forthcoming.

5. Daube, David: Transplantation: Acceptability of Procedures and Their Required Legal Sanctions, in G E W Wolstenholme and Maeve O'Connor, eds: *Ethics in Medical Progress: With Special Reference to Transplantation*, Ciba Foundation Symposium (Little, Brown & Co, Boston, Massachusetts) 1966.

6. Halley, M Martin, and Harvey, William F: Medical vs Legal Definitions of Death, *Journal of the American Medical Association*, vol 204, no 6, May 6, 1968, pp 423–425.

7. Kinsolving, Lester: in *The San Francisco Chronicle*, June 17, 1968.

8. Moore, Francis D: *Give and Take* (W B Saunders Co, Philadelphia, Pennsylvania) 1964.

9. *The New York Times*, June 8, 1968.

10. *The New York Times*, Aug 5, 1968, p 1.

11. *The New York Times*, Aug 10, 1968.

12. *The New York Times*, Aug 11, 1968, News of the Week in Review.

13. Reinhold, Robert: in *The New York Times*, Aug 5, 1968.

14. Schmeck, Harold M, Jr: *The Semi-Artificial Man: A Dawning Revolution in Medicine* (Walker & Co, New York, New York) 1965.

15. Starzl, T E: discussion of J E Murray: Organ Transplantation: The Practical Possibilities, in G E W Wolstenholme and Maeve O'Connor, eds: *Ethics in Medical Progress: With Special Reference to Transplantation*, Ciba Foundation Symposium (Little, Brown & Co, Boston, Massachusetts) 1966.

16. Stickel, Delford L: Organ Transplantation in Medical and Legal Perspectives, *Law and Contemporary Problems*, vol XXXII, no 4, Autumn 1967.

17. Thielicke, Helmut: Ethical Problems of Modern Medicine, unpublished lectures given at a conference on medicine, morals, and technology at the Institute of Religion, Texas Medical Center, Houston, Texas, Mar 25–28, 1968.

3.

A DEFINITION OF IRREVERSIBLE COMA:

REPORT OF THE "AD HOC" COMMITTEE OF THE HARVARD MEDICAL SCHOOL, UNDER THE CHAIRMANSHIP OF HENRY K. BEECHER, M.D., TO EXAMINE THE DEFINITION OF BRAIN DEATH

OUR PRIMARY purpose is to define irreversible coma as a new criterion for death [1]. There are two reasons why there is need for a definition: (1) Improvements in resuscitative and supportive measures have led to increased efforts to save those who are desperately injured. Sometimes these efforts have only partial success so that the result is an individual whose heart continues to beat but whose brain is irreversibly damaged. The burden is great on patients who suffer permanent loss of intellect, on their families, on the hospitals, and on those in need of hospital beds already occupied by these comatose patients. (2) Obsolete criteria for the definition of death can lead to controversy in obtaining organs for transplantation.

Irreversible coma has many causes, but *we are concerned here only with those comatose individuals who have no discernible central nervous system activity.* If the characteristics can be defined in satisfactory terms, translatable into action — and we believe this is possible — then several problems will either disappear or will become more readily soluble.

More than medical problems are present. There are moral, ethical, religious, and legal issues. Adequate definition here will prepare the way for better insight into all of these matters as well as for better law than is currently applicable.

CHARACTERISTICS OF IRREVERSIBLE COMA

An organ, brain or other, that no longer functions and has no possibility of functioning again is for all practical purposes dead.

Our first problem is to determine the characteristics of a *permanently* nonfunctioning brain.

A patient in this state appears to be in deep coma. The condition can be satisfactorily diagnosed by points 1, 2, and 3 to follow. The electroencephalogram (point 4) provides confirmatory data, and when available it should be utilized. In situations where for one reason or another electroencephalographic monitoring is not available, the absence of cerebral function has to be determined by purely clinical signs, to be described, or by absence of circulation as judged by standstill of blood in the retinal vessels, or by absence of cardiac activity.

1. *Unreceptivity and Unresponsitivity.* There is a total unawareness to externally applied stimuli and inner need and complete unresponsiveness — our definition of irreversible coma. Even the most intensely painful stimuli evoke no vocal or other response, not even a groan, withdrawal of a limb, or quickening of respiration.

2. *No Movements or Breathing.* Observations covering a period of at least one hour by physicians is adequate to satisfy the criteria of no spontaneous muscular movements or spontaneous respiration or response to stimuli such as pain, touch, sound, or light. After the patient is on a mechanical respirator, the total absence of spontaneous breathing may be established by turning off the respirator for three minutes and observing whether there is any effort on the part of the subject to breathe spontaneously. (The respirator may be turned off for this time provided that at the start of the trial period the patient's carbon dioxide tension is within the normal range, and provided also that the patient had been breathing room air for at least ten minutes prior to the trial.)

3. *No Reflexes.* Irreversible coma with abolition of central nervous system activity is evidenced in part by the absence of elicitable reflexes. The pupil will be fixed and dilated and will not respond to a direct source of bright light. Since the establishment of a fixed, dilated pupil is clear-cut in clinical practice, there should be no uncertainty as to its presence. Ocular movement (to head turning and to irrigation of the ears with ice water) and blinking are absent. There is no evidence of postural activity (decerebrate or other). Swallowing, yawning, vocalization

are in abeyance. Corneal and pharyngeal reflexes are absent.

As a rule the stretch of tendon reflexes cannot be elicited: i.e., tapping the tendons of the biceps, triceps, and pronator muscles, quadriceps and gastrocnemius muscles with the reflex hammer elicits no contraction of the respective muscles. Plantar or noxious stimulation gives no response.

4. *Flat Electroencephalogram.* Of great confirmatory value is the flat or isoelectric EEG. We must assume that the electrodes have been properly applied, that the apparatus is functioning normally, and that the personnel in charge is competent. We consider it prudent to have one channel of the apparatus used for an electrocardiogram. This channel will monitor the ECG so that, if it appears in the electroencephalographic leads because of high resistance, it can be readily identified. It also establishes the presence of the active heart in the absence of the EEG. We recommend that another channel be used for a noncephalic lead. This will pick up space-borne or vibration-borne artifacts and identify them. The simplest form of such a monitoring noncephalic electrode has two leads over the dorsum of the hand, preferably the right hand, so the ECG will be minimal or absent. Since one of the requirements of this state is that there be no muscle activity, these two dorsal hand electrodes will not be bothered by muscle artifact. The apparatus should be run at standard gains 10μv/mm, 50μv/5 mm. Also it should be isoelectric at double this standard gain which is 5μv/mm or 25μv/5 mm. At least ten full minutes of recording are desirable, but twice that would be better.

It is also suggested that the gains at some point be opened to their full amplitude for a brief period (5 to 100 seconds) to see what is going on. Usually in an intensive care unit artifacts will dominate the picture, but these are readily identifiable. There shall be no electroencephalographic response to noise or to pinch.

All of the above tests shall be repeated at least 24 hours later with no change.

The validity of such data as indications of irreversible cerebral damage depends on the exclusion of two conditions: hypothermia (temperature below 90° F [32.2° C] or central nervous system depressants, such as barbiturates.

OTHER PROCEDURES

The patient's condition can be determined only by a physician. When the patient is hopelessly damaged as defined above, the family and all colleagues who have participated in major decisions concerning the patient, and all nurses involved, should be so informed. Death is to be declared and *then* the respirator turned off. The decision to do˙ this and the responsibility for it are to be taken by the physician-in-charge, in consultation with one or more physicians who have been directly involved in the case. It is unsound and undesirable to force the family to make the decision.

LEGAL COMMENTARY

The legal system of the United States is greatly in need of the kind of analysis and recommendations for medical procedures in cases of irreversible brain damage as described. At present, the law of the United States, in all 50 states and in the federal courts, treats the question of human death as a question of fact to be decided in every case. When any doubt exists, the courts seek medical expert testimony concerning the time of death of the particular individual involved. However, the law makes the assumption that the medical criteria for determining death are settled and not in doubt among physicians. Furthermore, the law assumes that the traditional method among physicians for determination of death is to ascertain the absence of all vital signs. To this extent, *Black's Law Dictionary* (fourth edition, 1951) defines death as

> The cessation of life; the ceasing to exist; *defined by physicians* as a total stoppage of the circulation of the blood, and a cessation of the animal and vital functions consequent thereupon, such as respiration, pulsation, etc. [italics added].

In the few modern court decisions involving a definition of death, the courts have used the concept of the total cessation of all vital signs. Two cases are worthy of examination. Both involved the issue of which one of two persons died first.

In *Thomas* vs. *Anderson,* (96 Cal App 2d 371, 211 P 2d 478) a California District Court of Appeal in 1950 said, "In the instant case the question as to which of the two men died first was a question of fact for the determination of the trial court. . . ."

The appellate court cited and quoted in full the definition of death from *Black's Law Dictionary* and concluded, ". . . death occurs precisely when life ceases and does not occur until the heart stops beating and respiration ends. Death is not a continuous event and is an event that takes place at a precise time."

The other case is *Smith* vs. *Smith* (299 Ark, 579, 317 SW 2d 275) decided in 1958 by the Supreme Court of Arkansas. In this case the two people were a husband and wife involved in an auto accident. The husband was found dead at the scene of the accident. The wife was taken to the hospital unconscious. It is alleged that she "remained in coma due to brain injury" and died at the hospital seventeen days later. The petitioner in court tried to argue that the two people died simultaneously. The judge writing the opinion said the petition contained a "quite unusual and unique allegation." It was quoted as follows:

That the said Hugh Smith and his wife, Lucy Coleman Smith, were in an automobile accident on the 19th day of April, 1957, said accident being instantly fatal to each of them at the same time, although the doctors maintained a vain hope of survival and made every effort to revive and resuscitate said Lucy Coleman Smith until May 6th, 1957, when it was finally determined by the attending physicians that their hope of resuscitation and possible restoration of human life to the said Lucy Coleman Smith was entirely vain, and

That as a matter of modern medical science, your petitioner alleges and states, and will offer the Court competent proof that the said Hugh Smith, deceased, and said Lucy Coleman Smith, deceased, lost their power to will at the same instant, and that their demise as earthly human beings occurred at the same time in said automobile accident, neither of them ever regaining any consciousness whatsoever.

The court dismissed the petition as a *matter of law*. The court quoted *Black's* definition of death and concluded,

Admittedly, this condition did not exist, and as a matter of fact, it would be too much of a strain of credulity for us to believe any evidence offered to the effect that Mrs. Smith was dead, scientifically or otherwise, unless the conditions set out in the definition existed.

Later in the opinion the court said, "Likewise, we take judicial notice that one breathing, though unconscious, is not dead."

"Judicial notice" of this definition of death means that the court did not consider that definition open to serious controversy; it considered the question as settled in responsible scientific and medical circles. The judge thus makes proof of uncontroverted facts unnecessary so as to prevent prolonging the trial with unnecessary proof and also to prevent fraud being committed upon the court by quasi "scientists" being called into court to controvert settled scientific principles at a price. Here, the Arkansas Supreme Court considered the definition of death to be a settled, scientific, biological fact. It refused to consider the plaintiff's offer of evidence that "modern medical science" might say otherwise. In simplified form, the above is the state of the law in the United States concerning the definition of death.

In this report, however, we suggest that responsible medical opinion is ready to adopt new criteria for pronouncing death to have occurred in an individual sustaining irreversible coma as a result of permanent brain damage. If this position is adopted by the medical community, it can form the basis for change in the current legal concept of death. No statutory change in the law should be necessary since the law treats this question essentially as one of fact to be determined by physicians. The only circumstance in which it would be necessary that legislation be offered in the various states to define "death" by law would be in the event that great controversy were engendered surrounding the subject and physicians were unable to agree on the new medical criteria.

It is recommended as a part of these procedures that judgment of the existence of these criteria is solely a medical issue. It is suggested that the physician in charge of the patient consult with one or more other physicians directly involved in the case before the patient is declared dead on the basis of these criteria. In this way, the responsibility is shared over a wider range of medical opinion, thus providing an important degree of protection against later questions which might be raised about the particular case. It is further suggested that the decision to declare the person dead, and then to turn off the respirator, be made by physicians not involved in any later effort to transplant organs or tissue from the deceased individual. This is advisable in order to avoid any appearance of self-interest by the physicians involved.

It should be emphasized that we recommend the patient be declared dead before any effort is made to take him off a respirator, if he is then on a respirator. This declaration should not be delayed until he has been taken off the respirator and all artificially stimulated signs have ceased. The reason for this recommendation is that in our judgment it will provide a greater degree of legal protection to those involved. Otherwise, the physicians would be turning off the respirator on a person who is, under the present strict, technical application of law, still alive.

COMMENT

Irreversible coma can have various causes: cardiac arrest; asphyxia with respiratory arrest; massive brain damage; intracranial lesions, neoplastic or vascular. It can be produced by other encephalopathic states such as the metabolic derangements associated, for example, with uremia. Respiratory failure and impaired circulation underlie all of these conditions. They result in hypoxia and ischemia of the brain.

From ancient times down to the recent past it was clear that, when the respiration and heart stopped, the brain would die in a few minutes; so the obvious criterion of no heart beat as synonymous with death was sufficiently accurate. In those times the heart was considered to be the central organ of the body; it is not surprising that its failure marked the onset of death. This is no longer valid when modern resuscitative and supportive measures are used. These improved activities can now restore "life" as judged by the ancient standards of persistent respiration and continuing heart beat. This can be the case even when there is not the remotest possibility of an individual recovering consciousness following massive brain damage. In other situations "life" can be maintained only by means of artificial respiration and electrical stimulation of the heart beat, or in temporarily bypassing the heart, or, in conjunction with these things, reducing with cold the body's oxygen requirement.

In an address, "The Prolongation of Life" (1957) [2], Pope Pius XII raised many questions; some conclusions stand out: (1) In a deeply unconscious individual vital functions may be maintained over a prolonged period only by extraordinary means. Verification of the moment of death can be determined, if at all, only by a physician. Some have suggested that the moment of death is the moment when irreparable and overwhelming brain damage occurs. Pius XII acknowledged that it is not "within the competence of the Church" to determine this. (2) It is incumbent on the physician to take all reasonable, ordinary means of restoring the spontaneous vital functions and consciousness, and to employ such extraordinary means as are available to him to this end. It is not obligatory, however, to continue to use extraordinary means indefinitely in hopeless cases. "But normally one is held to use only ordinary means — according to circumstances of persons, places, times, and cultures — that is to say, means that do not involve any grave burden for oneself or another." It is the church's view that a time comes when resuscitative efforts should stop and death be unopposed.

SUMMARY

The neurological impairment to which the terms "brain death syndrome" and "irreversible coma" have become attached indicates diffuse disease. Function is abolished at cerebral, brain-stem, and often spinal levels. This should be evident in all cases from clinical examination alone. Cerebral, cortical, and thalamic involvement are indicated by a complete absence of receptivity of all forms of sensory stimulation and a lack of response to stimuli and to inner need. The term "coma" is used to designate this state of unreceptivity and unresponsitivity. But there is always coincident paralysis of brain-stem and basal ganglionic mechanisms as manifested by an abolition of all postural reflexes, including induced decerebrate postures; a complete paralysis of respiration; widely dilated, fixed pupils; paralysis of ocular movements; swallowing; phonation; face and tongue muscles. Involvement of the spinal cord, which is less constant, is reflected usually in the loss of the tendon reflex and all flexor withdrawal or nocifensive reflexes. Of the brain-stem-spinal mechanisms which are conserved for a time, the vasomotor reflexes are the most persistent, and they are responsible in part for the paradoxical state of retained cardiovascular function, which is to some extent independent of nervous control, in the face of widespread disorder of cerebrum, brain stem, and spinal cord.

Neurological assessment gains in reliability if the aforementioned neurological signs persist over a period of time, with the additional safeguards that there is no accompanying hypothermia or evidence of drug intoxication. If either of the latter two conditions exists, interpretation of the neurological state should await the return of body temperature to normal level and elimination of the intoxicating agent. Under any other circumstances, repeated examinations over a period of 24 hours or longer should be required in order to obtain evidence of the irreversibility of the condition.

REFERENCES

1. The *Ad Hoc* Committee includes Henry K Beecher, MD, *chairman;* Raymond D Adams, MD; A Clifford Barger, MD; William J Curran, LLM, SMHyg; Derek Denny-Brown, MD; Dana L Farnsworth, MD; Jordi Folch-Pi, MD; Everett I Mendelsohn, PhD; John P Merrill, MD; Joseph Murray, MD; Ralph Potter, ThD; Robert Schwab, MD; and William Sweet, MD.
2. Pius XII: The Prolongation of Life, *Pope Speaks,* vol 4, no 4, 1958, pp 393–398.

4. ETHICAL ISSUES IN EXPERIMENTAL MEDICINE

by M. H. Pappworth

CONSENT

Two facts concerning the problem of experimental medicine stand out above all others: namely, consent, and do ends justify means?

Undoubtedly, in experiments on humans, consent has become a broken reed. There is every reason to suspect that too often genuine consent is not obtained even in those cases where the experimenters claim otherwise. Consider some of the categories mentioned in my book, *Human Guinea Pigs* [9], such as the delirious, the comatose, the psychotic, and infants. Thirty-nine experiments of doubtful ethics done at Hammersmith Hospital are mentioned in that book, and in thirteen of them the patients used were infants and the very old, the delirious, the comatose, and those dying from malignant diseases. Did all these victims or their relatives give genuine consent?

In a review of *Human Guinea Pigs* in the *New Law Journal* the view was expressed that

> It is this question of consent and not whether this piece of evidence or that is reliable which has to be faced up to as a result of Dr. Pappworth's book. Why is the patient's consent not sought? If the answer is that it would not be forthcoming, clearly that is an answer whose implications are wholly damning. If the answer is that doctors would not wish to reveal the scope and nature of experimentation by seeking the patient's consent to it, even though consent might be forthcoming, in many instances, that is damning too [10].

The definition of consent was dealt with at great length by a British High Court Judge, Sir Roger Ormrod, in an address given to The Royal College of General Practitioners in November, 1967. Five quotations from his speech are very informative.

> The field can be narrowed a good deal further by the law of trespass — that is, it is an actionable wrong to interfere bodily with another person without his consent in the absence of clear therapeutic indications. This raises a dilemma which has been the playground of jurists for centuries and which looks like becoming a medical nightmare in the twentieth century — "when is consent not consent?"

> But in practice and in the individual case it is not very difficult to decide whether someone has or has not effectively consented. Judges and juries manage to do it many times a year. If the consent has been obtained by trick the law will treat it as no consent; on the other hand, failure to provide all the relevant information will not necessarily invalidate it.

> In certain special cases where one party is in a peculiarly weak position in relation to the other the law requires *uberrima fides* — that is, good faith and disclosure of all relevant facts. The relation of doctor and patient is one of these. Underlying the law's approach is the presumption that in general people over 21 are grown up and must take their own decisions. The law is not concerned with the motives or even the pressures which lead to their decisions unless the latter are so severe as to overwhelm their minds.

> He [the patient] will be entitled to demand a bona fide statement in broad terms of the risks to life or future health or of pain and discomfort involved in the contemplated procedure or to a frank admission that in the given circumstances these cannot be assessed with any accuracy.

> The greater the risk the greater will be the obligation on the doctor to insure that the patient understands [7:9–10].

I have talked personally to many doctors during the past twelve months specifically about explanations given to patients by them or their seniors when seeking consent for experimentation. I am amazed how often the real scope of the experiment is not divulged, and yet the experimenters claim that they have sought and obtained consent and say so in their medical publications. For example, I have often been informed that many experimental physicians, when seeking consent for cardiac or liver catheterization, even for the most complex multiple procedures, tell patients merely that a tube or catheter is to be inserted into a blood vessel of their arm or leg (or both), but do not inform the patient that the catheter will be further passed far beyond its point of insertion, possibly along the femoral artery, through abdominal aorta via the pelvic arteries, and then through the thoracic aorta of the chest, and so through the left ventricular chamber of the heart, and that, indeed, two or even three such catheters may be passed at the same time into the various heart chambers, a long, long way from their point of insertion. Does this conform with the views of consent elaborated by Judge Ormrod?

An important Canadian law case is relevant and may be a salutary warning to experimentalists who purposely avoid proper explanations. An engineering student submitted himself as the subject of a test involving the administration of a new anaesthetic agent. The experiment was done at the University of Saskatchewan and the plaintiff was paid fifty dollars for taking part in the experiment (such compensation is a common procedure in America and Canada). During the experiment the plaintiff's heart stopped and in order to restart it the doctors opened his chest in order to massage his heart manually. After the heart had stopped for one and a half minutes it restarted, but because of the temporary lack of oxygen to his brain induced by the cardiac arrest, he remained unconscious for four days. Subsequently he complained that his memory had become poor and his concentration impaired. He was awarded $22,500 and this was upheld, with costs, at a subsequent court of appeal.

In their judgment, the judges maintained that although the appellants had told the plaintiff that an incision would be made in his arm and that a catheter or tube would be inserted into his vein, they did not inform him that the catheter would be advanced into and through his heart until it became positioned in his pulmonary artery. By withholding that information, "informed consent" had not been obtained and the appellants had been guilty of trespass. The judges further stated that

> The subject of medical experimentation is entitled to a full and frank disclosure of all the facts, probabilities and opinions which a reasonable man might be expected to consider before giving his consent, and the question of risks being properly hidden from a patient when it is important that he should not worry can have no application in the field of research [4].

Special consideration regarding consent must apply to patients dying, especially from incurable diseases. Two different types of research on such patients can be readily differentiated: 1) experiments which might possibly benefit the individual, and 2) experiments which have no direct relationship with the patient's own personal illness.

The first category of experiments includes the use of drugs, surgical procedures, and non-conventional radio-therapy which might inhibit the progress of the malignant condition. But even then the ethical issues are not clear cut, because a person who thinks that he is dying and is told that an experiment might possibly help him or even somebody else is likely to agree to anything, however drastic or mutilating. In fact, this may be only another form of coercion, the patient being blackmailed by his fear of death. An expert on cancer, Dr. T. B. Brewin of Glasgow, wrote to me, highlighting another dilemma with this group of patients.

> I have found that one of the most difficult problems is the grateful trusting, poorly educated patient, who does not want and whose anxiety will be positively increased by a detailed explanation of all that is involved, including what might happen. Is it right to rely on their trust that you will not go too far, and to dispense with the explanations and the details?

With regard to experiments which have no relevance to the actual disease inflicting such patients, a statement made at the Council for International Organizations of Medical Sciences is worth quoting. The speaker was Professor Alfred Gellhorn of Columbia University, and he expressed the view

> that no form of experiment was justifiable on the basis that the patient was going to die anyway — such experiments on the "hopeless case" might eventually diminish the doctor's concern for human life. If the patient is moribund no useful conclusions could be derived from any results, while, if he was not, how could the doctor be certain of the hopelessness of the position [2]?

Some Canadian doctors did the following experiment. A woman was deeply comatose due to liver failure. A 67-year-old man with inoperable lung cancer agreed to the experiment. A catheter was passed in each of these patients via the umbilical (navel) vein into the portal (liver) vein and another catheter was passed in each of them via the femoral (thigh) vein into a major pelvic vein. The free end of each of these four catheters was connected to a mechanical pump so that the man's blood was channeled into the recipient's (the woman's) pelvic veins and so into her liver veins and from there was driven through the man's liver, where it was hoped that the toxic substances which should have been dealt with by the woman's liver would be destroyed, and into his general circulation and then removed via his pelvic veins back into the recipient in a continuous circuit [14]. The experiment was a failure, but concerning it *World Medicine* commented editorially,

> But is it realistic for doctors to talk about such a patient making a totally free choice in the light of all the facts? When does explanation become persuasion, and choice become obligation? And do the persuasive arguments even need to be formulated in words for them to be appreciated by a patient [11]?

A further interesting point about consent was raised specifically concerning the work on experimental measles vaccine [see

9:57]. The administrators of the hospital protested vigorously against the inclusion of that experiment in my book, maintaining that they had had consent from the parents. Leaving aside the important issue whether any parent has the moral right to submit his or her child to unpleasant experiments, another important issue developed. It subsequently transpired that the parents of six of the children used in the experiment did not reply to the written request for consent. These children were considered to be "abandoned," and the physicians took upon themselves the responsibility for using them in the experiment. Ministers of Health, in their defense of experimental medicine, have often pointed out that patients who consider themselves to have been maltreated in hospital have the protection of the law. But these mentally defective children could not possibly bring an action against anybody by themselves, and nobody can bring an action on their behalf. The legal validity of the hospital's assumption of guardianship and their rights and duties towards "abandoned children" have never been defined. When questioned in 1967, the Minister of Health agreed that the matter was one of urgency, but twelve months later he has not yet given a decision. Matters concerning the National Health Service are outside the sphere of activity of the present ombudsman. The public should clamor for the rectification of this glaring anomaly.

With regard to those people who volunteer to have experiments performed upon them, an interesting observation was made at Harvard Medical School. It was shown that over 60% of such volunteers were maladjusted and had problems in adapting themselves to their social environment [1]. Other inquiries have confirmed that such volunteers may, from a psychological point of view, differ considerably from the rest of the population. This further complicates the problem of consent. Indeed, there are a few eccentric people, sometimes psychotics, who are so masochistic that they submit themselves to needless operations and even mutilations. Are they to be encouraged and their mental peculiarity exploited in the interests of medical science?

DO ENDS JUSTIFY MEANS?

I believe that experimental physicians never have the right to select martyrs for society. They should be utterly condemned when they are activated, even to the slightest degree, by a desire for prestige, acclaim, or promotion. As long as promotion and success in the medical profession continue to depend on published research, there will always be those few who are unscrupulous enough to do anything to gain personal preferment.

Whether an experiment gained its desired results or not is to me immaterial. Two British professors of medicine have both declared that although they themselves would not have had the temerity to have been among the first to have performed certain procedures such as liver puncture or combined right and left heart catheterization, they both imply that we should not now criticize these innovators but be thankful for the benefits their experimental boldness bestowed upon mankind, even though their pioneer work may have caused much suffering and even death. To me, this is casuistry at its worst, because it condones false ethical standards. An experiment is ethical or not at its inception, and does not become so *post hoc* because it achieved some measure of success.

An example of this peculiar reasoning took place on a live television program I did with Dr. Fletcher of the Hammersmith Hospital. After I had briefly recounted the experiment done in his hospital [9:128] and challenged him to justify it, he replied that the investigator was young and enthusiastic at the time. But that person is still young and enthusiastic and actively engaged in research. Two of the first deaths directly due to liver puncture done by Professor Sheila Sherlock were on "moribund patients," one of whom was a man of 75 with general paralysis of the insane who also had inoperable bowel cancer with widespread secondaries [15]. No doubt by that man's death she improved her technical skill and possibly our knowledge, but did the end justify the means? Professor Sherlock herself has written, "Needle biopsy of the liver should be regarded as potentially fatal. A real indication for its use must always be present" [12:291]. Every human being has the right to be treated with decency and that right belongs to each and every individual and should supersede every consideration of what *may* benefit mankind, what *may* contribute to the public welfare, what *may* advance medical science. No doctor is justified in placing science or the public welfare first and his obligation to his patient second. Any claim to act for the good of society should be regarded with extreme distaste and even alarm, as it may be a high-flown expression to cloak outrageous acts. A worthy end does not justify unworthy means.

CODES OF CONDUCT

The most famous code regulating the ethical conduct of doctors is the Hippocratic Oath, which was formulated about 400 B.C. But its wording and some of its content are not acceptable today, and doctors are no longer required to take this oath before admission to the profession. After the Nuremberg trial of the infamous Nazi doctors, the judicial tribunal with the help of expert doctors formulated a new code of conduct. The World Medical Organization on several occasions has reformulated and amended these rules to satisfy various criticisms and objections; the last rewriting was in 1964. But no government ever declared these rules to be mandatory on their doctors.

It is not a sufficient safeguard to patients to leave the whole matter of the conduct of experiments to the conscience of the individual doctors as has often been stated as official policy. In our modern Freudian permissive society, doctors, like many others, claim to be the sole judge of their own conduct and brook no interference, regarding rules as infringements of their freedom. The Book of Judges records that one of the most disastrous periods of Jewish history was when "Every man did that which was right in his own eyes." Such an attitude by doctors and medical administrators may lead to tragic happenings. The medical profession by itself is not competent to draw up any code because science alone cannot supply adequate and trustworthy principles. Religious leaders and those thoroughly acquainted with the principles of moral philosophy must be consulted and their advice heeded. The Churches, the Law, and Parliament must express their opinions collectively and state how much further they are prepared to allow the medical profession to take risks with human lives in order to achieve possible advances in knowledge. Sir Roger Ormrod expressed the following opinions about codes of ethics for experimental physicians:

> The primary function of a code of professional ethics is to adjust the balance of power so as to protect the patient or client against the practitioner who has the immense advantages which are derived from knowledge and experience.
>
> A secondary but no less important function of a code of ethics is to protect the main body of practitioners who comply with its provisions against exploitation by the black sheep who are prepared to defy them [7:7–8].

SOME VIEWS EXPRESSED AT THE COUNCIL FOR
INTERNATIONAL ORGANIZATIONS OF MEDICAL SCIENCE

This organization was set up by UNESCO and the World Health Organization, and the conference was held in Paris in October, 1967, and reported fully in the UNESCO magazine *Courier* [5]. Sir John Eccles of Chicago (formerly of Australia), who won the Nobel Prize in Medicine in 1963, described experiments done by others in the United States on a large number of mental patients. Multiple trephine holes were made in the skull of each patient and through each hole electrodes were inserted into the brain. These electrodes were left in place for many months, and at regular intervals electric currents were passed through them and the effects on the patients' actions and behavior noted. Sir John described the resultant brain damage as "fantastic" and further said,

> . . . in relation to investigations which are of a dubious, or to my mind, unallowable, kind, that a great proportion of these investigations could be satisfactorily done in primates; . . .

When you say that you fully explain something to the subject, telling him what the lesion is or what he is going to be subjected to, and he gives his consent, I do not believe in the case of the brain that you can explain what you are going to do, because none of us knows sufficient about the brain to be able to say to a subject simply, precisely and with assurance that this is all that it will do.

Other opinions expressed at this conference include the following:

In Austria therapeutic experiments are permitted in university clinics, but the law forbids them in other hospitals. Thus the patient admitted to a university hospital knows that new procedures not yet in current use may be used for his benefit. This being the case, it is unnecessary to inform him fully; nor is it possible when a new procedure is being utilized. . . . It is undesirable that the patient should know everything, and that is indeed the problem involved in his being informed of a trial to be carried out on him. (Theodor Brücke, Professor of Pharmacology, University of Vienna.)

Experiments on healthy people are an entirely different matter. . . .
The great danger must be pointed out of sacrificing human beings on the altar of science and glorifying subjects who volunteer to be guinea-pigs. . . .
I shall say nothing about the clinical trials that have been carried out on prisoners condemned to death or on civil prisoners in for a term of years. To me they seem to be contrary to the moral concepts of the human person. (Robert de Vernejoul, Professor of Medicine, Paris.)

It may be of interest to point out that British law in general is very permissive with respect to the use of human subjects in scientific study while it is highly restrictive with regard to the use of animals. This great interest in animal welfare is not limited to Great Britain. In the United States today, for example, no popular national movement exists to lobby for regulation of clinical investigation on human subjects, while at least three very well-supported national organizations are clamoring for additional legislation to regulate animal experimentation. (Maurice B. Visscher, Professor of Physiology, University of Minnesota, Minneapolis.)

I have the feeling that there is a great deal of duplication going on at the moment in clinical investigation. . . . The planning of clinical investigation should be submitted to a review by a knowledgeable body of experts in the particular field involved. And duplication of human experimentation should be avoided if possible, at least within one country, and later if possible in the whole world. (Alexis de Muralt, Professor of Physiology, University of Berne, Switzerland.)

ORGAN TRANSPLANTATIONS

Experimental organ transplantation in animals has gone on for over 50 years with varying success and consequent varying enthusiasm. It has been shown during the past decade that the plumbing aspect of such surgery is not only feasible but can be carried out successfully. (By the plumbing aspect I mean the technique of removal of a diseased organ such as the kidney, heart, liver, or lungs, and its replacement by an organ from a human [live or dead] or an animal.) This success is spectacular and a virtuoso triumph acclaimed with fanfares of praise and ballyhoo by the mass media of press, radio, and television.

But the great problem of rejection has not been overcome. This refers to the fact that the body possesses powerful defense mechanisms (immunological reactions) against the entry into the body of any foreign material. In particular, the white blood corpuscles play an important role in this defense mechanism. One of the end results of these natural defense processes is that tissue grafted into people from an animal or other human is destroyed (rejected) by the host.

In the case of corneal transplants such rejection is least likely because the cornea is normally comparatively avascular (with a poor blood supply), so that only small amounts of the protein substances produced by the white blood cells in order to neutralize and reject the incursion of the foreign substance actually reach the cornea, and so its survival is very likely. But with other organs like the heart, which have a very abundant blood supply, rejection will occur.

Ways have been devised to overcome this rejection by interfering with the development and immunological activities of the white blood cells. This has been attempted with some success by the combined use of drugs such as azathioprine (which is toxic to the bone marrow), steroid drugs (which have many undesirable side effects), irradiation, and, more recently, the experimental antilymphocytic serum, the value of which has yet to be proven. But nature exhorts a severe price for all this unnatural and severe onslaught against the body's natural defense mechanisms. More than anything else, the patient's resistance to all types of infections is also, as a direct consequence of this treatment, greatly reduced and this is often the immediate cause of death after transplantation. But it is illogical and misleading to boast, as has been done in several transplant cases, that the patient did not die because of tissue rejection but from an infection. If he had not been given these powerful and toxic materials to combat rejection, he would not have succumbed to the infection, so the unresolved problem of safely combating rejection was really the cause of his death. Moreover, any patient who has received an organ transplant, other than a cornea, will have to take some drugs to suppress his immune reactions in an attempt to prevent future rejection of the transplant. He will thereby be subjected to the inconveniences, the psychological disturbances, and the potential toxic effects of these drugs. Above all, he will always be liable to a markedly increased susceptibility to infection, and what would be a minor illness in a normal person may become an overwhelming infection, probably fatal, in such a patient.

Experimental work indicates that with vascular organs rejection *always occurs* sooner or later. What cannot be predicted is the duration of apparent acceptance of the transplanted organ, whether that will be days, weeks, months, or years. Moreover, the unpredictable length of this period may be much shorter in fact than the recipient's life expectancy without transplantation. It is also claimed that the risks of transplantation surgery, however great, are justified because the prognosis otherwise is hopeless. But hopeless in terms of weeks, months, or years cannot be accurately foretold by any doctor. No doctor, however skilled or experienced, can precisely balance the expected period of survival without transplant with the period before which organ rejection becomes complete, an interval which is itself unpredictable. Experienced physicians have seen many patients survive, for example, from chronic cardiac failure for several years without being restricted by total incapacity. The South African transplant expert, Dr. Christiaan Barnard, at a meeting of the American College of Cardiology in March, 1968, rejected the argument that there is no certainty as to how long such a patient may live and stated that what is more important to the physician is "how the patient is going to live." But his most successful heart transplant, although he has survived for over six months, is still capable of only minor physical activity.

DONOR SOURCE

Another great problem is the source of the donor organ. Though some surgeons still persist in transplanting animal organs into humans (livers from pigs, hearts from chimpanzees, among others), the invariable lack of success, which from an immunological consideration would appear to be inevitable, has caused all but a very few, I think misguided, surgeons to abandon this practice.

It is only with a paired organ such as the kidney that a live donor is possible. Live donors have been and still are used for kidney transplants, but the prospective donor is rarely a truly free agent [9:171]. Other actual occurrences have been: 1) A young woman in the late stages of pregnancy was persuaded to be a donor. 2) A man was exhorted, "You cannot let your colleague down and let him die." But after he had donated his kidney he was surprised that an insurance company would not accept him as a first class life. He felt that he should have been warned prior to his sacrifice. 3) A donor was discovered on a chest X-ray immediately prior to the removal of his kidney to have active pulmonary tuberculosis, but the surgeon did not inform him of this and did not initiate treatment until after he had seized his kidney.

The public has also been frequently misled by radio, press, and television giving far too optimistic figures of likely success in renal transplants. Certainly better results have been achieved during the past two or three years, but survivals for over four years are still likely to be very few and a success rate of 75% which has sometimes been claimed cannot be substantiated and is extremely misleading.

There are ethical and legal problems concerning the use of cadavers as a source for organ transplantations. Unless the organ is removed soon after death and used almost immediately, it is liable to have undergone rapid deterioration resulting from lack of oxygen, because blood is no longer circulating through it. This very important time factor is at most four hours for a kidney but only about half an hour for a heart. It is indefensible to transplant a damaged organ (because of inadequate oxygenation of its tissues) into a recipient, because the transplanted organ, even if it is not rejected soon, is unlikely to function adequately, and the patient and his relatives have been misled by false hopes and promises of likely success. But some enthusiastic surgeons have done just this, presumably attempting to make the best of a bad job. If transplant surgery is carried out, then the material used must be the best possible. It is also for this reason that donors should be young. A large percentage of those past middle age have at least minor disease of the blood vessels of their organs, probably as a normal concomitant of body aging processes. Such organs will not be 100% healthy. However well intentioned, it is futile for those above the age of forty to offer to donate their organs, other than a cornea, for transplants when they die.

It follows from this that the best source of cadaver donor material is from a young person who is unlikely to have any disease or vascular involvement of heart, lungs, kidneys, or liver. This limits the potential source of donors to young people who have died from brain lesion (either severe injury or tumor). But a further problem is that such brain damaged patients may remain comatose for weeks, months, or even years before they die. It is not my purpose to discuss the ethics of strenuously trying to keep such comatose patients alive, remaining like cabbages, unresponsive to their surroundings, incapable of communication or locomotion, which is often done.

However, as a potential transplant donor, the longer the patient is comatose the longer his kidneys, heart, lungs, and liver are likely to suffer from inadequate circulation and thus not be ideal material for the purpose. The tremendous dilemma therefore arises that those youngsters with brain damage are ideal donors only if the period of coma prior to removal of their organs is short. But is it justifiable either morally or legally to shorten purposely the "twilight zone" prior to actual death?

This problem has brought into the open the question of defining death. Until recently this was not considered to be a problem at all, and cessation of heartbeat and breathing were the accepted criteria (conventionally the duration of cessation of these functions should be five minutes before death is pronounced by the doctor [3]. But machines have been devised which can take over the mechanics of breathing and circulation. Thus, when a young person is admitted to the hospital after a severe head injury or with an inoperable brain tumor, doctors know from experience that undoubtedly such a patient's life span is limited, but nobody can say with certainty whether he will live without medical intervention for hours, days, weeks, months, or even years (in the case of head injury). If he is connected with a mechanical apparatus his breathing and circulation can be maintained indefinitely, although he will still remain comatose. When a suitable patient for an organ transplant is admitted the doctor can then turn off the machine which has been keeping the comatose patient alive, thus stopping the heart and respiration, and then immediately remove the wanted organs. By his action, the doctor determines the actual time and mode of death of the donor. It has been admitted that some surgeons, in their endeavor to get the wanted organs in the best possible condition, have removed them from the comatose patient even prior to turning off the machine.

Concerning this the legal correspondent of the *British Medical Journal* wrote:

> It may have happened very occasionally that vital organs have been removed for the purpose of transplantation from the body of a comatose patient thought to be dying. Persons responsible for such surgery would be in danger of criminal proceedings. To ask consent of the next-of-kin would be no defense if criminal proceedings were to be initiated. Indeed the request for consent is likely to raise such a mental conflict for the next-of-kin, already under some stress, that the making of the request itself is of doubtful ethical morality [6].

Some doctors have claimed that such action is justifiable because the older concepts of recognizing the actual time of death are obsolete. They claim that an absence of demonstrable electrical activity of the brain, shown on an electroencephalogram (EEG) should be the criterion even though the patient's heart is still beating and he is still breathing. The absence of such electrical activity is presumed to indicate irreversible brain damage such that only a "cabbage" existence is possible. But will doctors who are not transplant enthusiasts and will lay and church leaders and Members of Parliament agree to this new definition of death?

Even if this definition is accepted, many problems still remain. For how long should the absence of electrical activity be recorded before death is certified? This is very controversial. Some experts claim that 48 hours is a necessary period, but others would be satisfied with a much shorter time. But cases have been recorded of patients not only surviving after even longer periods of absence of electrical brain activity than 48 hours, but even regaining consciousness. Professor Pierre Soulié, a Parisian cardiologist, has reported the case of a 17-year-old boy who, while undergoing surgery for a congenital heart lesion of comparative minor severity (a patent ductus) had cardiac arrest followed by complete absence of electrical brain activity shown on an EEG which lasted for 6 days. Yet this boy made a complete recovery and is now working for his baccalaureate [13]. So we cannot accept this suggested criterion of death without reservation.

Dr. Pampiogne, England's leading authority on electroencephalography, has condemned the use of that technique in any spurious attempt to define or determine death. The argument against its use has been further emphasized by a report from the Royal Infirmary Edinburgh on five comatose patients (due to poisoning) who had no EEG responses for periods up to eleven hours, and yet four of them made a complete recovery with no residual physical or mental damage.

Moreover, EEG recording and interpretation are both very highly skilled tasks; there are few in Britain capable of expert opinion on such matters, and very few British hospitals have the services of such an expert. But much of this discussion is merely academic, because those transplant surgeons who have availed themselves of comatose brain damaged donors have rarely used an EEG machine to determine the moment of death, but have relied on "clinical judgment" that the brain damage was such that the patient could not survive for long except possibly in a "cabbage" state and was beyond surgical help.

A chronological account of the first human heart transplant makes gruesome reading [8]. It was done at the Groote Schuur Hospital, Cape Town, Republic of South Africa, on December 3, 1967, under the direction of Dr. Christiaan N. Barnard. At 4 p.m. a young woman was knocked down by a car and sustained multiple fractures and severe head injuries, and soon afterwards was admitted comatose to the hospital, where she was treated for shock by supportive measures for her circulation. At 9 p.m. it was decided to transfer her to the cardio-thoracic unit of the hospital as a potential heart donor. At 10 p.m. she was connected with a mechanical respirator. At that time her heart action as shown by electrocardiograph was normal. A neurosurgeon declared that her brain damage was such that surgery would be to no avail and the head injury would undoubtedly prove lethal. At 12:45 a.m. she was removed to the operating theatre, the artificial lung ventilation being continued. Meanwhile, because of treatment, her blood pressure had risen from the very low value of 60 mm to 100 mm, indicating a marked improvement in her circulation. At 2:20 a.m. the respirator machine was deliberately turned off and at 2:32 a.m. cardiac arrest was reported; at that moment an incision in her chest was made and her heart removed. The picture of a surgeon hovering over a dying patient ready to snatch her organs is a ghoulish one. The transfer of a patient from one hospital ward to another (in some cases there has been such a transfer from one hospital to another) and then to an operating theatre adjoining one in which the recipient is being prepared is apparently a necessary procedure, but it is profoundly distasteful.

A great deal of publicity has been given to allegations by certain British surgeons that their transplant work was being hindered by the stringencies of the 1961 Human Tissues Act. A potentially or actually fatal accident case admitted to the hospital might be a suitable donor for organ transplant, but delay in getting permission from the next of kin might vitiate against successful transplant. Permission should also be invariably obtained from the coroner, since legally the body of anybody dying from unnatural causes belongs to him, and this is likely to cause further delay. Actually, several transplants have been done illegally without asking the coroner's permission. If organs are removed without permission from either the next of kin or the coroner then the surgeon, under the present law, lays himself open to an action for trespass.

Sir Gerald Nabarro took up the surgeon's case in the House of Commons and introduced a Bill which surprisingly received an unopposed second reading on April 5, 1968. The Bill mentioned, "Permit to remove from the body of a human person, duly certified dead, kidney or kidneys required for medical purposes, unless there was reason to believe that the deceased during his lifetime had instructed otherwise." How the deceased could have possibly instructed anybody except during his lifetime is difficult to understand. More important, the phrase "duly certified dead" is too vague and the problem of the definition of death is completely evaded. Also objectionable is the principle that silence implies consent is not acceptable to many informed medical or lay people. The limitation of the Bill to kidney transplants is wholly illogical. Fortunately, H.M. Government refused to support the third reading of the Bill.

Transplant surgery raises still more issues. With our agreed shortage of resources in Britain is it justifiable to expend so much money, so much time, and such great talent on the possible benefit of a very few when so very many require less controversial, less spectacular, less dramatic, even humdrum surgery which has a much greater chance of success? Consider the fact that in some parts of Britain patients have to wait as long as two years for hospital admission for such a necessary operation as the repair of a hernia (rupture). The same applies to operations for enlarged prostate glands. Here there is the additional important point that when this is done as a planned operation the mortality is about 3%, but if it is delayed emergency surgery may become necessary, increasing the mortality to about 20%. Surely the greatest good should be available for the greatest number, taking into account the available resources. Such experimental innovations as transplant surgery must be seen in their proper perspective.

No surgery, including transplant surgery, should be done merely because it has been shown to be possible. In the past, patients with cancer have had the whole of the lower part of their body amputated, which is a terrific technical feat, and such patients have survived a few months. (Incidentally, would they have agreed to this if they had fully appreciated what it involved?) But feasibility alone should not be considered as justification for such heroics.

The public must not be misinformed about transplant surgery. It never cures the original disease or renders the recipient normal. The older the patient the more likely he will have vascular disease in other organs than the one removed. No organ of the body exists in complete isolation and independence of the other structures. For example, coronary disease, for which a heart transplant may be considered, is almost always associated with a generalized vascular disease involving all organs, and the same applies to most cases of kidney disease.

To how many transplants is it justifiable to submit any one individual? Many were upset by the news in July, 1968, that a second heart transplant was contemplated on the second Cape Town patient, and that possibly liver and lung transplants were to be done as well. Have the implications of all this been seriously considered by the surgeons? Have they the moral right to act as they think fit? Has the lay public the moral right to attempt to restrain them? Imagine a Hitler kept alive indefinitely by repeated organ transplants, although his diseased brain had gradually degenerated more and more. Will wealth and position determine who are going to be the recipients and who the donors? Imagine a battlefield strewn with casualties and ghoulish surgeons snatching organs from some of the dying and deciding who among the others will be kept alive by transplantations. All this is possible. Let us intervene before it is too late.

FINANCIAL ASPECTS OF HEART TRANSPLANTS

Some interesting figures have been published on the estimated costs of some of the much publicized heart transplants. Michael Kasperak, who was operated on at Stanford, California, lived for 15 days. The total cost was $28,845.83, which included $7,200 for blood at $25 per pint, $3,256 for the transfusions themselves, and $6,947 for the laboratory tests. The cost of Philip Blaiberg's initial 115 days in the hospital in Cape Town after his heart transplant was $34,300. The estimation of the cost of the first London heart transplant case, who survived 46 days, was $1,200 per day. None of these figures includes any surgical fees, which were waived in all cases.

REFERENCES

1. Florkin, Marcel: Medical Experimentation on Man, *The UNESCO Courier*, Mar 1968, pp 20–23.
2. Gellhorn, Alfred: in Experiments on Man, *British Medical Journal*, vol 4, Oct 14, 1967, p 105.
3. *Glaister Medical Jurisprudence*, 12th ed, 1966.
4. *Hlushka* vs *University of Saskatchewan, et al, Western Weekly Law Reports*, vol 52, 1965, p 609.
5. Medical Experimentation on Man: The Scientists Speak Up, *The UNESCO Courier*, Mar 1968, pp 24–27.
6. Moment of Death, *British Medical Journal*, vol 2, Aug 27, 1966, p 533.
7. Ormrod, Sir Roger: Medical Ethics, *British Medical Journal*, vol 2, Apr 6, 1968, pp 7–10.
8. Ozinsky, J: Cardiac Transplantation — The Anaesthetist's View: A Case Report, *South African Medical Journal*, vol 41, no 48, Dec 30, 1967, pp 1268–1270.
9. Pappworth, M H: *Human Guinea Pigs: Experimentation on Man* (Routledge & Kegan Paul Ltd, London, England) 1967; (Beacon Press, Boston, Massachusetts) 1968.
10. The Patient's Consent, *New Law Journal*, vol 117, no 5286, May 18, 1968, p 556.
11. A Really New Ethical Problem?, *World Medicine*, vol 3, no 10, Feb 13, 1968, p 9.
12. Sherlock, Sheila: Needle Biopsy of the Liver: A Review, *Journal of Clinical Pathology*, vol 15, 1962, pp 291–304.
13. Soulié, Pierre: in *Paris Match*, Jan 20, 1968.
14. Swift, J E; Ghent, W R; and Beck, I T: Direct Transhepatic Cross-Circulation in Hepatic Coma in Man, *The Canadian Medical Association Journal*, vol 97, no 24, Dec 9, 1967, pp 1435–1445.
15. Zamcheck, Norman, and Klausenstock, Oscar: Liver Biopsy (Concluded). II. The Risk of Needle Biopsy, *New England Journal of Medicine*, vol 249, Dec 24, 1953, p 1064.

5. THE ABORTION DEBATE

by Ralph B. Potter, Jr.

MANY individuals and groups in the United States want reform of the laws governing abortion. To gain political leverage, reformers must mobilize opinion within the massive Protestant community, for in the increasingly widespread political contests over abortion law reform the mainline Protestants generally constitute a "swing vote." What basic concepts shape Protestants' attitudes toward abortion? What arguments impress them?

Protestants traditionally have disapproved of the termination of any healthy pregnancy. Amidst the present ferment and strife, however, American Protestants are showing signs of confusion regarding the proper moral and legal status of abortion. Various streams of thought have been converging to form a theological and ethical blend which is eroding the inherited Protestant position of disapproving abortion in all circumstances in which the life of the mother is not seriously threatened.

BENEFITS OF THE STATUS QUO

The first clue to Protestant confusion is the extent of the silence of the churches on the question of abortion. No one knows the exact dimensions of the abortion problem, but it is a problem of no less significance than other matters on which the churches have invested great energies. The degree of uncertainty regarding the incidence of abortion in the United States is best illustrated by the conclusion of a distinguished committee which reported to a major conference on abortion, May 29, 1957:

> Taking into account the probable trend of the abortion ratio
> since the interwar period, a plausible estimate of the frequency

85

of induced abortion in the United States could be as low as 200,000 and as high as 1,200,000 per year, depending upon the assumptions made as to the incidence of abortion in the total population as compared with the restricted groups for which statistical data are available, and upon the assessment of the direction and magnitude of bias inherent in each series of data. There is no objective basis for the selection of a particular figure between these two estimates as an approximation of the actual frequency [6:180].

During the churches' participation in a variety of civic crusades in recent decades, the practice of nontherapeutic abortion has remained morally condemned and legally proscribed, but widely practiced and perennially ignored. How has it been possible for the churches not to address themselves to the reform of abortion laws which, according to advocates of "liberalization," presently drive a million women a year to endanger life and health at the hands of criminal abortionists, engender a criminal empire, corrupt law enforcement officials, discriminate against the poor, force the cultivation of deformed embryos, ensure the birth of unwanted children, deny women control of their own bodies, and perpetuate a bogus moralism and hypocrisy? It seems out of character for the heirs of the social gospel, who frequently find it difficult to suppress their passion for prefecting the social order, to abstain from correcting a situation considered grievous by many social critics. How can we account for this unusual reticence?

The best explanation appears unduly simple and circular: Protestants have been relatively content with the status quo. They seem to have concluded that it represents the best possible balance of their conflicting inclinations towards "law" and "grace." The untidy arrangement by which antiabortion laws are retained, but enforced only sporadically against criminal abortionists and never against their clients, has allowed Protestants to employ the didactic, educative power of the law to reinforce their strong negative judgment upon abortion itself; yet relief from the stringency of the rule is afforded in individual cases by tolerating the existence of a decentralized system of illegal abortion accessible to women equipped with the resources necessary for individual enterprise in any sphere — that is, motivation, information, and money. If the resulting inequities have been unattractive, the alternatives have seemed still less attractive. Enforcement of the law would forestall relief for "exceptional cases." A weakening of the law might imply an acceptance, in principle, of nontherapeutic abortion.

NEW RECEPTIVITY

The social education and action machinery maintained by the major Protestant denominations has not been mobilized in the battle for or against abortion law reform. But it is increasingly difficult for Protestants not to become embroiled, especially in those states in which bills providing for the extension of the justifiable grounds for abortion have been introduced in the legislatures in recent years.

New legislation extending the provisions for legal abortion was passed during 1967 in Colorado, North Carolina, and California. Extensive and well publicized controversy was occasioned by the introduction of an abortion law reform bill in the New York State legislature. The bill died in committee but gave public life to the abortion issue. Abortion law reform bills have been introduced in at least twenty-four other states.

Numerous groups have been formed to promote the cause of reform. (The Association for the Study of Abortion, centered in New York, conducts the most extensive program. The Association prepares and distributes pamphlets, bibliographies, and reprints, provides speakers, conducts forums, and promotes the gathering and exchange of information about abortion.) The audience attentive to these groups has expanded; the new resonance may be attributed not so much to any novelty in the message as to changes in the sensitivities of listeners. The main elements of the abortion issue are not new; zeal for reform is not new; most of the arguments are not new. It is the receptivity of a broad segment of the "Protestant" public that is new.

Three factors have contributed most to this new receptivity. The first is the breakdown of old theological certainties which shaped Protestant opposition to nontherapeutic abortion. What has broken down is a constellation of beliefs about nature, man, and God which sustained the conviction that nascent life in the womb is, in every circumstance, a gift of God given for the realization of his mysterious purpose, and is, therefore, to be respected as inviolable from lawful human interference except in the tragic case in which the life of the fetus is pitted against the life of its mother. Protestants seldom have relied upon the natural law reasoning of Roman Catholic theologians to sustain their disapprobation of abortion. Protestant objections generally have not been grounded in a desire to avoid intervention in the biological processes of "nature," and "nature" has not been invested with a sacral immunity from pragmatic human manipulation. Protestants have feared not an "abuse of nature" but rather a direct affront to "nature's God." Abortion has been viewed as the annulment of God's special providence, the ungrateful despising of his miraculous gift, and the rejection of his summons to the vocation of parenthood.

The Protestant approach has rested upon the prevalence of Providence. When a new habit of mind now attributes new life to "rotten luck" in the practice of contraception rather than to the purposeful will of a merciful God, neglect of the countermeasure of abortion becomes irrational and superstitious retreat from the possibility of exercising control of one's destiny. Denial of accessibility to abortion comes to be seen by many as a violation of a civil liberty.

The second factor underlying the new receptivity consists of the abortion reform movement's forceful expression of themes taken from the Protestant tradition itself, particularly the themes of self-determination and rational control of nature. The principle of self-determination vindicates the attempts of autonomous individuals to shape the conditions of their existence through vigorous action. It functions as a counterprinciple, offsetting the invitation to passive acceptance of the dictates of nature conveyed in the biologically bound version of natural law philosophy underlying Roman Catholic discourses on abortion. Rational control of nature is indispensable for the realization of self-determination. As the realm in which men acknowledge the providential rule of God contracts, the scope of human control must expand. Parenthood ought to be planned because such an important matter must be submitted to purposeful control. If men are unable to believe that God has carefully planned and ordained each pregnancy, they themselves must take measures to insure that procreation is not left to "blind nature" or to chance. The status of abortion is enhanced among Protestants when it is advertised as a means of implementing rational control over nature.

The third factor contributing to the new receptivity is the dimming of the vision of a Protestant American made to conform to the dictates of Protestant conscience. Reformers assert that control over nature is a moral imperative and frequently add that self-determination in the use of reproductive powers is a civil right. Protestants, convinced of the high value of control over nature and of self-determination, feel obliged, in a pluralistic society, to concede the exercise of these powers to all men. Those who disagree concerning the specific *content* of the imperatives of conscience must, nevertheless, be afforded the freedom necessary for self-determination through control over nature. By devotion to their own principles, Protestants are obliged to tolerate a gap between what is *morally* condemned and what is *legally* proscribed.

Protestants are confused concerning the *moral* status of abortion when practiced *by Christians*. Their confusion is compounded by uncertainty regarding the extent to which the moral judgments of one segment of society should be imposed upon *others* by *legal* enactment. The unpleasant aftertaste of Prohibition lingers on. More and more Protestants acquiesce to the motto, "You can't legislate morality." They concede that there must be a sphere of privacy into which the state and its law may not intrude. But does abortion fall within this sphere? Is abortion merely a matter of "private morality"? Are the existing laws regulating abortion simply relics of an antiquated paternalism which precludes the exercise of self-determination and restricts the area to be submitted to human control? Do our abortion laws serve only to reinforce a peculiar, religiously grounded code of moral behavior which has lost power to gain voluntary assent? Or, in a pluralistic society, can some valid secular purpose establish the propriety of legal restrictions upon the practice of abortion? These have come to be the decisive issues among Protestants now forced to reconsider their stance on abortion law reform.

THE SPECTRUM OF CONTENDING VIEWS

The rallying point for those intent upon reformation of the abortion laws is the relevant section of the Model Penal Code proposed by the American Law Institute [2; 17; 31]. The suggested code would justify a physician "in terminating a pregnancy if he believes there is substantial risk that continuance of the pregnancy would gravely impair the physical or mental health of the mother or that the child would be born with grave physical or mental defect, or that the pregnancy resulted from rape, incest, or other felonious intercourse." Support for this proposal has come from disparate sources, from individuals and groups who find themselves in an impromptu alliance with others with whom they may share no other cause or belief. Even supporters of less extensive modifications can be classified, with technical accuracy, as "advocates of abortion law reform." Such a broad label may be polemically useful to opponents of reform, but it obscures distinctions between many shades of opinion concerning how lenient the law should be and prevents recognition of the many different patterns of reasoning that are employed to support these varied opinions.

If rational debate is to be promoted, careful distinctions must be made along the broad spectrum of recommendations put forward concerning abortional law reform. The spectrum may be divided into three major segments, three broad bands marking fundamentally different approaches to the issue. At the right end of the spectrum is a position that may be awkwardly referred to as "no abortion." At the left end is "abortion on demand." Those who fall within the middle range of the spectrum support the concept of "justifiable abortion."

[The term "left wing" will be used to include some who occupy the left end of the middle segment of the spectrum, that is, those who would permit very generous indications but would still require that some "reason" be given in support of a request for a legal abortion. Similarly, the "right wing" includes many "fudging Catholics" who, although formally committed to the "no abortion" position by the Papal Encyclical, *Casti Connubi,* issued December 31, 1930, nevertheless manage to make allowance for action "to prevent pregnancy" after rape and condone laws which permit therapeutic abortion necessary to save the life of the mother. The necessity of providing a flexible boundary for the right wing is confirmed by proposals advanced by Robert F. Drinan, S.J., Dean of Boston College School of Law [12:177–179].]

In their style of argument, the members of the middle or "justifiable abortion" school differ from adherents of the two extreme positions by their willingness to require and to accept certain reasons or "indications" as adequate justification for the basically repugnant act of abortion. Within this middle school there is wide disagreement concerning which indications should establish acceptable grounds for abortion under the law. But all members agree that abortion may be justifiable for certain reasons and unjustifiable for other reasons. In contrast, neither of the extreme positions deals in reasons or "indications." Those who uphold the "no abortion" position deny that there is any reason that could render abortion morally and legally tolerable. Advocates of "abortion on demand" reject the notion that any reason should be required, since all decisions regarding the use of procreative powers must be left to the unrestricted private judgment of individual women. Debate over the identity of legally acceptable indications is thus properly a characteristic of the middle range of the spectrum. It is within this range that the immediately foreseeable compromises of the law will be hammered out.

Compromise is characteristic of the middle. An intellectual compromise determines the approach and the style of debate within the middle segment. Content is drawn from the left. But the framework which determines the structure of argumentation about the limits of "justifiable abortion" is a legacy of the style of moral theology that has flourished among Roman Catholics on the right. The intellectual framework of debate is similar in form to the apparatus employed by moral theologians in assessing the claim that a particular resort to armed force represents an instance of "justifiable warfare." The burden of proof is imposed upon those who would assert, in a particular case, that an exception should be conceded from the general condemnation and prohibition. It is ironic that Roman Catholics apply this apparatus in thinking about warfare but refuse to let it structure their thought upon abortion. Protestants rely upon it in debate concerning abortion but have neglected to make conscious use of it in the analysis of the moral problem of war. The motives for neglect have been similar in the respective cases: the framework provides an apparatus for the regulation rather than for the abolition of a particular type of activity. Protestants have harbored the hope of abolishing war; Roman Catholics would like to abolish abortion.

The traditional framework, with its generally negative judgment upon abortion, has determined the shape of the abortion law reform bills modeled upon the American Law Institute proposals. Moreover, public debate has, for the most part, conformed to the pattern of delineating the proper sphere of allowable exceptions. But the sphere is expanding. Under the present compromise new content is being squeezed into the form determined by the venerable framework. In response to considerations pressed most assiduously by secular humanists, whose basic affinity is with the "abortion on demand" school, the sphere of recommended exceptions has been inflated to the extent that the encompassing apparatus is distended nearly to the point of explosion and collapse.

The compromise that dictates that new, far-reaching extensions of the allowable indications be debated within a framework designed to restrict exceptions leads to curious adaptations of the traditional vocabulary. The "Statement of Policy" of the Society for Humane Abortion, a group disposed to the cause of abortion on demand, reveals a sensitivity to the prejudicial effect of the established framework of discussion: "Because we regard abortion as a surgical procedure and not a criminal offense, we neither endorse new laws nor sponsor revision of old laws which attempt to control abortions. The underlying concept of enacting such laws simply perpetuates the idea that abortion is wrong." Nevertheless, the same Statement conforms to the pattern of offering a list of justifying indications for abortion. Even so, the list itself reveals that the conformity is a tactical, rhetorical device which conforms to the style imposed by the framework in order to subvert its strictures.

> Be it therefore resolved that the Society for Humane Abortion supports abortion for those wishing to terminate pregancy if:
> 1. There would be grave impairment of physical or mental health of the pregnant woman
> 2. Pregnancy resulted from failure of birth control devices or through ignorance of their use
> 3. Pregnancy resulted from rape or incest
> 4. The child would probably be born with a serious physical or mental defect
> 5. There exists *some other compelling reason* . . . physical, psychological, mental, spiritual or economic [36].

A resolution adopted by the Unitarian Universalist Association in 1963 parallels this statement, omitting the second item but preserving verbatim item five.

THE LEFT WING: ABORTION ON DEMAND

The further one moves to the left along the spectrum, the stronger is the inclination to treat self-determination as an absolute value. It is the master theme in a medley of arguments drawn from a variety of sources. An argument for abortion on demand is likely to be composed of the following elements arranged in differing patterns of emphasis. Abortion on demand is necessary: (1) to protect the life and health of women by making medically safe abortion available to those who cannot be deterred by rigid laws or high risks; (2) to preserve the autonomy of the medical profession; (3) to insure that only wanted children will be born; (4) to guarantee that each child will receive careful nurture within a family able to expend adequate amounts of time, money and loving care upon it; (5) to help defuse the population explosion; (6) to enable women to attain equal status through escape from the risk of unwanted pregnancy; (7) to avoid discrimination by race and social class through making abortion equally available to all at low expense; (8) to realize the promise of full civil liberty by according women unquestioned control over the use of their bodies, and couples unchallenged right of privacy [29; 18].

These themes are variously elaborated and supplemented; but they are invariably accompanied by strong emphasis upon the right of self-determination as a positive moral value which can be realized only through repeal of laws which presume to prescribe who may and who may not legally terminate her pregnancy. The central significance of the moral value of self-determination is illustrated in a passage written by Thomas S. Szasz:

I submit that efforts to "liberalize" abortion laws by providing a broader spectrum of medical and psychiatric justifications for the procedure are, in effect, restrictive of human freedom and, therefore, truly anti-liberal. Why? Because medical and psychiatric "liberalizations" of abortion laws would only increase the number of times *other* people could provide abortions for women; they would not increase the number of occasions on which women could make this decision for *themselves*. Such measures, therefore, give assent to the proposition that it is good to deny people the right to determine for themselves how they should use their bodies [37:344].

Such an argument finds new receptivity among Protestants exposed to theological works which assure them that "Christian ethics aims, not at morality, but at maturity" [23:54].

Many younger Protestants have been nurtured in the certainty that maturity is exhibited in the willingness to accept moral ambiguity and the risk of the exercise of freedom in each new situation. Presently fashionable styles of thought simultaneously corrode the ancient tradition and create a new affinity for the major positive themes voiced by advocates of abortion on demand. (In the opening chapter of *Situation Ethics*, Joseph Fletcher illustrates the alleged benefits of the freedom and flexibility afforded by his "situational approach" to ethics by showing how it might be used to justify abortion in certain circumstances [15:37–39]. Paul Ramsey notes with irony that, "Even in *Situation Ethics* one comes upon at least one general rule of behavior, or general principle of ethics, besides love itself. . . . That rule is: '. . . no unwanted or unintended baby should ever be born.' Or, to express this for a *subject* other than the child: no woman should be forced to bear an unwanted child" [32:168].)

These intellectual currents run so wide and deep that it is certain that the present legal and political contests focused upon the American Law Institute proposals for "justifiable abortion" represent only an initial phase of an inevitable conflict between the demand for unhampered self-determination and the tradition which asserts that there is a valid basis for public regulation of the practice of abortion. The impact of the left-wing school is strong enough that one may anticipate a significant shifting of the burden of proof. In many quarters, the central question of the abortion debate is gradually being rephrased. The question becomes: "What reasons can justify the refusal of the state to grant permission for an abortion?" The form of the question preserves the style of the middle; but the content reveals the influence of the left. Eventually, the question must be faced, "Why should there be any law governing who may undergo an abortion?"

THE RIGHT WING: REALIZATION OF THE GREATER GOOD

The right wing of the spectrum is defended most relentlessly in public debate by Roman Catholic spokesmen. It should not be overlooked, however, that some members of the Protestant and

Jewish communities join in defense of the present laws regulating abortion. Nevertheless, most of the right-wing arguments stated here are to be attributed to Roman Catholic commentators who, by and large, have set the terms of debate over and against left-wing advocates.

As one moves toward the right end of the spectrum, certainty increases that it is the proper function of the state to intervene in the matter of abortion in order to prevent harm. The harm envisioned may be inflicted upon the mother, the medical profession, the family, society at large, the fetus, or what might best be described as "the cultural ethos."

The nub of the right-wing argument, as presented to contemporary Americans, is simple and stark: the condoning of widespread resort to abortion would undermine civilization. The argument is couched in theological terms; it leads, however, to conclusions in the realm of cultural anthropology. The path of reasoning sometimes twists through philosophical thickets. But the destination is a flat prediction concerning consequences for all human relationships if a significant number of people come to accept abortion in good conscience. There are many distractive bypaths along the route to be traversed in argument. But the constant goal is to convince hearers, by whatever arguments carry force in their generation, that the practice of abortion is incompatible with the attainment of man's true humanity. At stake in controversies over abortion law reform is the definition of the vision of what man should be. Urgency arises from the conviction that the content of that vision will shape the actual quality of human relationships in decades to come.

The profundity of the right-wing argument is its greatest weakness. Many of the injuries described by controversialists on the right take place in a dimension of existence unknown or unexplored by their fellow citizens. Indeed, when the particular "harms" are analyzed closely, they are seen to consist ultimately of a deprivation of a greater good, a good which may transcend the concern of a secular, pluralistic state. Can the prevention of such a harm, or the realization of such a good, be considered a valid legislative purpose sufficient to overrule the strong desires of innumerable pregnant women? Analysis of the difficulties experienced by right-wing critics in dramatizing the injuries they presume to be wrought upon mothers by abortion will suggest the perils of profundity and illustrate the dynamics of the abortion debate.

The harm that is most vivid and imaginable to typical onlookers is injury to the health and welfare of the mother. Spokesmen for the left wing generate great dramatic impact by portraying very palpable injuries to mothers. They depict vivid harm to victims with whom readers can readily identify. The power of immediacy is exploited also in their outline of causes and cures. The harm is attributed directly to the lack of legal access to medically competent abortions performed in hospital settings. A prompt remedy is offered through "legalization of abortion now." In the effort to recoup the title of "defenders of the public welfare," right-wing advocates are obliged, by contrast, to depict either very subtle injuries to real persons or somewhat less subtle harm to less vividly imaginable entities such as "society," "civilization," or "the fetus." Indeed, the attempt to overcome the seeming inability of many people to visualize the fetus as an object of real injury accounts for many of the intellectual and rhetorical maneuvers in the battle over abortion law reform.

Both the left and the right wings of the abortion spectrum would like to enjoy a reputation as guardians of the life and health of mothers. But how are life and health truly protected? Members of the left wing join with many moderates of the middle segment in urging that permission for abortion should be granted when the measure is deemed necessary by physicians to spare a woman from a nonlethal threat to her health. Going beyond that, the left wing emphasizes the need to protect women from the risk to life and health incurred through criminal abortion. The right wing asserts that true life and health are best served by guarding women from abortion in any circumstance.

To reinforce its claim to be the true guardian of the mother, each side provides empirical data concerning the incidence of abortion, both legal and illegal, and the medical and psychiatric effects of abortion performed under various circumstances. The left wing must overcome public inertia. Its spokesmen are compelled to show that a massive problem exists that ought not to be ignored. Hence, their estimates of the incidence of criminal abortion tend to be high. Moreover, their statistics must indicate that criminal abortions are very dangerous while hospital abortions are medically safe and seldom give rise to untoward psychological effects.

Conversely, statistics presented by the right wing diminish the danger gap between hospital and extrahospital abortions. Emphasis is placed by right-wing spokesmen upon the residual risk of the operation under even the best medical conditions. It is asserted that "sound medical practice" would require abortion only in exceedingly rare circumstances. With the advance of medical skill, strictly medical indications have been reduced. It is rare that life or health is seriously jeopardized in well attended pregnancy. Moreover, it is claimed, there is no strong evidence of significant therapeutic gain through abortion. There is a lack of due proportion between the undoubted risk and the uncertain gain.

The right wing's first line of defense — that abortion, as a medical procedure, is both dangerous and superfluous — seems to be crumbling under an avalanche of statistics from Eastern Europe and other regions where abortion is widely practiced and new techniques are being developed through research. The level of medical danger there is not high. Also, it can be argued that abortion is not totally superfluous. If it is seldom necessary, abortion may nevertheless be occasionally necessary, and the law should not bar physicians from attempting to preserve the life and health of their patients.

There is a second line of defense. The dangers of abortion may be more subtle. The unhappy effects may be delayed in time and buried in the recesses of the personality, accessible only to those armed with psychiatric skill. Many on the right wing insist that, no matter where, or by whom, or for what reason abortion is performed, it inflicts a scar upon the conscience of the woman and places her mental health in jeopardy by exposing her to the harsh retribution of guilt.

A considerable body of literature deals with the psychiatric effects of abortion. From this literature adherents of the left wing extract evidence that the incidence of serious psychological after-effects is relatively low. They go on to argue that the incidence would be much lower still if right-wing propaganda did not per-petuate the self-fulfilling prophecy that induces symptoms of guilt by contending that such symptoms are virtually inevitable. They hold that guilt over abortion is a cultural legacy that will become increasingly rare as societies adopt a more "enlightened" and therefore more tolerant attitude toward abortion.

The reply of those on the right wing is to make the injury from abortion appear more subtle still. They hold that some psy-chiatrists cannot detect the full extent of the harm to mothers because they maintain a superficial view of the full components of true health. True health involves more than "a state of com-plete physical and mental wellbeing." It has a spiritual dimen-sion. The injury to the spirit of one who violates the law of nature and commandment of God by indulging in abortion may escape the notice of observers who employ less sensitive indices of affliction.

The depth of the disagreement which leads to strikingly dif-ferent estimates of how harm to mothers is to be avoided comes clearly into view in debate over the meaning and function of guilt. All agree that women should be spared the experience of guilt. The left would remove the cultural inducement to exhibit this learned response. Adherents of the right wing insist that the only way to be rid of guilt is to avoid the occasion of guilt. In their view, guilt is not simply a legacy from an unenlightened past. It is a sign of latent health, a danger signal that the law of nature cannot be violated with impunity. Given the reality of abortion as the extermination of innocent life for self-centered purposes, women *ought* to feel guilty. Indeed, the *absence* of guilt is a grievous symptom which reveals that callousness and spiritual sclerosis are far advanced. Women should be spared the occasion of guilt by the refusal of abortion. But, if abortions are to be performed, the entire community must be saved from experiencing a *lack* of guilt.

The third line of defense of the right-wing claim to be the true guardian of women is the claim that the practice of abortion frustrates the realization of man's true humanity. Evidence for this is not easily given. It is difficult to muster "hard empirical data" to convince those who, on other bases, do not already share a particular view of men. The difficulty exposes the true nature of the dispute and demonstrates the burden of profundity.

With regard to the protection of mothers, as on other issues, participants in the abortion controversy talk past one another. Reformers on the left gather statistics which purport to prove that, at least in certain nations, few women experience deep remorse after an abortion. But the statistics, even if acknowledged as accurate, have little effect upon right-wing commentators. Their arguments are not grounded in such observations. Their line can be defended with the aid of statistics that show abortion *does* have ill effects. But it cannot be overthrown by empirical evidence that abortion does *not* have bad medical or psychiatric consequences. Only the outer defenses can be endangered by the attack of epidemiologists and sociologists. The inner defense is founded firmly upon theological ground. The battle is being fought over questions of theological anthropology and ethics. The issue is: What ought man to be? What style of life represents the realization of true humanity?

HIGH STAKES

The central claim of the right wing is that abortion is evil because it deprives an individual of the greater good of becoming a more selfless creature. Abortion, in killing the actual self of the fetus, kills the potential higher self of the mother. Abortion is inimical to the attainment of "a generous spirit" which welcomes new life and accepts the occasion of redemptive suffering and sacrifice.

At stake in the abortion debate is not simply the fate of individual women or even the destiny of individual nations and cultures. It is difficult to demonstrate that acceptance of the most extreme proposal for abortion on demand would establish a clear and present danger to the civil harmony necessary for the maintenance of a tranquil state. Nations that have lenient abortion laws do function. But if abortion is not an actual threat to minimal public order, it may nevertheless be a symbolic threat to the ideal moral order espoused by Christians for two millennia. Abortion does not merely contradict specific mores and moral teachings pertaining to sexuality, marriage, and procreation or endanger a system of law built upon "respect for life." It implies the rejection of a world view which has sustained a way of life, a mode of being in the world, a pattern of response to the human condition.

Abortion is a symbolic threat to an entire system of thought and meaning. The willingness to practice abortion, or even to condone resort to abortion by others, signals that the high Christian vision of selfless charity has become despised and rejected of men. The Christian portrayal of the true man as one characterized by selflessness, sacrifice, concern for the weak and the unlovely, and a willingness to accept and transcend allotted afflictions through the power of redemptive suffering has faded in public consciousness to the point that it can seldom induce willing imitation. For many people there is simply no meaning in putting up with an unwanted circumstance when recourse is available without a high probability of temporal retribution.

For Christians, an entire system of meaning may be at stake in the abortion debate; but is anything at stake for a secular, pluralistic state?

SOURCES OF THE ABHORRENCE OF ABORTION

Christians frequently are delighted to take credit for instilling into the Western tradition a deep abhorrence of abortion. This affirmation of the historical relevance of Christianity may do wonders for Christian pride and morale, but it makes it more, rather than less, difficult to maintain antiabortion laws in a secular, pluralistic setting. Norman St. John-Stevas, a British Roman Catholic barrister and member of Parliament, has celebrated the role attributed to Christian faith in the emergence of respect for the fundamental value of "the right to life."

> The respect for human life and personality that distinguishes Western society from the totalitarian societies of the East did not spring up out of nothing. It is deeply rooted in experience and history. Above all it is rooted in religion. Ultimately the idea of the right to life, as is the case with other human rights, is traceable to the Christian doctrine of man. . . . The value of human life for the Christian in the first century A.D., as today, rested not on its development of a superior sentience but on its unique character of the union of body and soul, both destined for eternal life. The right to life thus has a theological foundation. . . . Respect for the lives of *others* because of their eternal destiny is the essence of the Christian teaching. Its other aspect is the emphasis on the creatureliness of man. Man is not absolutely master of his own life and body, he has no *dominion* over it but holds it in trust for God's purposes.
>
> This respect for human life has become part of the moral consensus of Western society [34:16, 17].

By this account, a ban on abortion might seem to be a particular application of the fundamental principle ascribed to Christian influence. But St. John-Stevas suggests that the sentiments which lead to sanctions against abortion have a more general source.

> This attitude to young life undoubtedly has in part a Christian foundation but it goes back beyond the Christian era to earlier civilizations. Rejection of abortion seems to result from the nature of man himself. . . . With the coming of Christianity condemnation of abortion was reinforced and became absolute [34:36].

Is the rejection of abortion really rooted in the nature of man himself? Or does it derive from a response to the image of man portrayed in the Gospels? The issue cannot be settled by available anthropological data which seem to indicate a general ambivalence towards the practice of abortion within societies which differ greatly in the rate of occurrence and the severity of the sanctions imposed [8:97–152; 9].

The more emphasis is placed upon the distinctively Christian roots of the ban on abortion, the more difficult it becomes to argue that the restrictions can or should be maintained if the theological roots from which they sprang have now been eroded. St. John-Stevas observes that the concept of the right to life "is accepted by many who would reject the Christian doctrine on which it is based." But he implies, nevertheless, that the pillars of Christian faith are necessary props for the ban upon abortion: ". . . the right to life is ceaselessly challenged. . . . Against these attacks the Christian doctrine of man, as a being destined for eternal life, and therefore of unique value, provides the most effective bulwark" [34:127]. An increasingly shaky popular belief in man's eternal destiny is, in these days, an unsteady foundation for domestic legislation.

It seems credible that Christian apologists are correct in the historical judgment that the harsh condemnation of abortion expressed in our laws is the precipitate of Western exposure to Christian moral teaching. An evangelical vision of how men ought to behave has been imposed as the legal norm of how they must behave. The requirements of love have been confused with the demands of natural justice.

In an extensive law journal article, Eugene Quay provides an example of the extent to which Christian expectations of self-sacrificing charity have crept into Roman Catholic definitions of conduct to be required by legal enactment.

> A mother who would sacrifice the life of her unborn child for her own health is lacking in something. If there could be any authority to destroy an innocent life for social considerations, it would still be in the interests of society to sacrifice such a mother rather than the child who might otherwise prove to be normal and decent and an asset [30:234].

Willingness to sacrifice one's health for the sake of an unborn child would seem to many people to represent an heroic achievement rather than a minimal gesture necessary to qualify one as "an asset" to society. Quay's rendition of the natural law and the nature of man has been skewed by Christian norms; the model of charity has been taken as the mandate of the law.

Through the teaching of the church, the faithful may come to look upon self-sacrifice as "normal and decent." It is difficult to convince the unfaithful, who may not share the prior conviction that man should be something more than he is, that abortion makes man something less than he ought to be. The mother who refuses to sacrifice her health may be "lacking in something," but that something is superadded to the level of morality that the state must require in order to preserve its stable existence.

The teaching of the church generated the sentiments expressed through the ban upon abortion. Abortion is a practice which seems incongruous with the profession of faith of those who live under the sign of the cross. But the nation does not live under the sign of the cross. Why, then, should there be laws restricting abortion? Do such statutes serve any secular purpose which may invest them with binding force in a society no longer willing to submit to the tutelage of the church?

WHAT VALUES DO ABORTION LAWS PROTECT?

The harm attributed to abortion by right-wing critics of legal reform is subtle and profound; it is the deprivation of man's greatest good — a character formed by charity and humble obedience to the commandments of God. But the very nobility of the vision places it beyond the protective concern of the law.

The state cannot command charity, but it can enforce justice. If it could be demonstrated that abortion did injury to some proper subject of the law's protection, a more solid foundation for antiabortion statutes could be constructed. This is the challenge to the right wing and to the middle: they must indicate a harm the law cannot ignore to a victim the law is bound to protect. The Christian commentator is goaded by a moral abhorrence of abortion derived from the charitable lesson of the Gospel. But to defend public laws against abortion he needs legal arguments derived from the universal norms of natural justice.

LATENT FUNCTIONS OF THE LAW

Society must have an appropriate and adequate reason for denying a woman legal access to a medical procedure she desires, oftentimes with great desperation. The protection of all men from the loss of the high moral stature considered by some to constitute man's greatest good is not, in itself, a suitable basis for restrictive legislation. What reasons can be given for such laws?

Left-wing spokesmen insist that the original intent of the American laws passed in the nineteenth century was to protect the prospective mother from the medical dangers of abortion which, given the state of medical art at that time, were extremely high [22:97]. Now, as medical skill has increased, the same motive requires revision of the statutes so that women who cannot be deterred by the persuasion of counseling or the threat of law can have abortions in the safety of the hospital under excellent medical care. Right-wing historians hold that the intention of the law has been to preserve the life of the unborn child and that this purpose remains a valid and sufficient basis for laws restricting abortion, for example, Quay: "Protecting the life of the unborn child has been a major concern of the earliest laws known to us. It has continued to be an object of lawmaking in every subsequent civilization which has contributed to our own because it springs from a universal feeling which in the past has ceased to move men only when a nation was in decay" [31:395].

The compromise established by the present laws realizes neither intention fully. The laws fail to deter women from risking life and health at the hands of criminal abortionists and, in failing to deter mothers, they fail to preserve the lives of the unborn children. Why then do the laws persist? Edwin Schur has searched for an answer to this sociological puzzle.

> Since present abortion laws have clearly failed to curb the un-sanctioned termination of pregnancy, their persistence must be attributable to some latent function they serve for society as a whole or for certain groups and individuals [35:59].

He suggests that every social system must maintain its member-ship; hence, "no society has allowed uncontrolled termination of pregnancies. . . . It may be also that the members of our society feel some illusory satisfaction in maintaining a formal and ideal standard in this area, even if they are largely unable to con-form to it" [35:59]. For Schur, "It is not even clear, however, just what the normative ideal embodied in present abortion laws represents." He mentions the possibility that "the proscription basically represents a direct prohibition on killing the fetus" [35:60]. But he gives greater attention to the assumption that the ban flows from the intention to prohibit illegitimacy and promiscuity or from "the insistence that woman shall not with ease voluntarily renounce motherhood as a major social role. . . . This could be interpreted as an institutionalized support of the 'maternal instinct,' a necessary sex division of labor, or a rein-forcement of the subordinate social status of women" [35:60].

Portions of Schur's analysis can be bolstered and refined by close scrutiny of data from public-opinion polls. Alice Rossi's presentation and interpretation of data gathered in a National Opinion Research Center poll in December 1965 [33] can be extended to undergird the theory that public attitudes towards abortion laws can best be explained by viewing them in the light of the traditional vision of the Christian family. The vision de-picts a family, faithfully trusting Providence, living as a pro-creative unit within which all parental sexual activity is channeled and confined.

In the Rossi data, the level of public acceptance of abortion varies sharply with the circumstances surrounding pregnancy. The more the circumstances and the reaction of the mother can be interpreted as being congruent with the ideal of the faithful procreative family, the greater is the measure of popular assent. Public reaction to the most frequently urged "indications" for abortion is recorded in Table 1.

TABLE 1
ATTITUDES TOWARD LEGAL ABORTION [33:36]
1482 respondents

"Please tell me whether or not you think it should be possible for a pregnant woman to obtain a legal abortion. . . ."

	Yes	No	Don't Know
If the woman's own health is seriously endangered by the pregnancy	71%	26%	3%
If she became pregnant as the result of rape	56	38	6
If there is a strong chance of serious defect in the baby	55	41	4
If the family has a very low income and cannot afford any more children	21	77	2
If she is not married and does not want to marry the man	18	80	2
If she is married and does not want any more children	15	83	2

The preservation of the life and health of the mother is an important precondition of the welfare of any family. Yet when the mother's health is at stake one quarter of the respondents disapprove of abortion. Even the weightiest considerations cannot overcome for some respondents the conviction that willingness to sacrifice the life of the unborn is incompatible with the "generous spirit" which must pervade the model family. As the benefits allegedly to be gained through abortion become less indispensable to the very existence of the ideal family, the rate of disapproval of abortion increases.

The belief that a mother should voluntarily accept her role provides a point of leverage for the argument that she need not accept the involuntary pregnancy imposed upon her by rape.

The norms derived from the vision of the ideal family clash dramatically when there is a serious risk of deformity. The desire to complete the family circle with the birth of a healthy, normal child is respected. Yet the refusal to be reconciled to the prospect of bearing and rearing a handicapped child violates the expectation of trust in Providence and in the power of the faithful to redeem and transcend adversity. When the same argument is lodged against the economic indication, it is not met by such a formidable counterprinciple. The level of public acceptance of abortion declines sharply at this point. As for the unmarried mother, interpretation of the NORC data would suggest that those imbued with the vision of the ideal family look upon her as one attempting to sever all the links which bind sexual intercourse, procreation, and family responsibility. The implied function of sex becomes recreative rather than procreative or unitive.

Few people in the NORC sample approve of the use of abortion as a means of birth control within marriage. Yet married women, unwilling at the moment to bear a child, constitute the largest segment of the clientele of criminal abortionists. This awkward fact is frequently skirted by reformers of moderate middle persuasion. Public reluctance to grant the healthy married woman's request for abortion cannot be accounted for convincingly by theories — frequently invoked in the case of the unwed mother — which center upon the repressed hostility of the pious toward sexual license. Nor can the condemnation be attributed to the belief that sex must never be purposefully separated from procreation, since there is evidence of widespread acceptance of contraception among those who would refuse abortion. An explanation consonant with our theory is that most people feel that the existence of a new life, or a potential new life, establishes a value and creates a presumption against abortion. The married woman who can produce no reason for her child not to be born other than her own unwillingness to receive it, seems to despise that potential life by sacrificing it to nothing more than her own convenience. Her refusal to accept the residual risk of pregnancy in marital intercourse is taken by many respondents to reveal a stubborn and selfish spirit incompatible with the generous adaptability which must sustain the true family.

THE PRESERVATION OF INDIVIDUAL CHARACTER

In order to provide a secular purpose for the legislative restriction of abortion, those sharing the inclinations of the right wing can argue that the ban on abortion functions not simply to uphold a particular code of behavior, let alone a peculiar code of sexual behavior. It upholds character, the type of character that is indispensable to good citizenship. The virtues necessary to sustain the true family are the virtues necessary to sustain the state. The virtues and vices exposed in dealing with matters of sex, family life, and procreation pervade the entire character and find expression in civic relations. The state has a stake in the promotion of self-restraint rather than self-indulgence, responsibility rather than irresponsibility, and selfless adaptability rather than selfish rigidity.

There is more to this phase of the argument than the cry that acceptance of abortion will lead to sexual promiscuity. The fear is rather that it will lead to a general decline of individual character through lax enforcement of responsibility. The issue is not whether sex is to be separated from procreation, but whether procreation can be divorced from the responsibility to nurture new life.

Most commentators at every point across the spectrum might be willing to concede that in American society, by and large, sex has already been separated from procreation. This can be accomplished, with fair reliability, by practice of the rhythm method, which is cheap, simple, available without reliance upon a supplier, and is well advertised in literature widely distributed by the Roman Catholic Church. The new sexual mores that may evolve will doubtless be labeled "promiscuous" by some moralists and welcomed by others. In either case, it is too late to suppress the knowledge that, except for occasional "accidents," sexual intercourse need not result in procreation. The small but enduring margin of error gives rise to the question, "Who will bear the risk of contraceptive failure?"

Right-wing commentators insist that the woman must bear the residual risk of pregnancy because her dismissal from that responsibility would bring on a widespread eagerness to evade every troublesome inconvenience which members of society must bear. To this, critics reply that the desire to escape the "natural consequences" of our actions is not only common and in most circumstances approved; it is, in fact, the stimulus to research and progress. The progress attained by permitting abortion as an emergency backstop to contraception would be the upgrading of parenthood and the realization of a happy family in a home in which every child would be wanted and welcomed. Men applaud the extension of human control into all other areas. Advocates of reform ask, "Why should this one act be set off as inaccessible to control?" The answer from the right wing is that life is present. No matter how tenuous the existence of a newly formed embryo, its creation is an event of moral import that cannot be totally ignored or despised.

The battle line is drawn at the point at which the relentless extension of self-determination and control over nature collides with the fundamental principle of "respect for life." Should there be no limit to willful manipulation, no inclination to concede that there are boundaries to the power that may safely be entrusted to men? The fear expressed by the right wing is that if the law does not contest a woman's claim that she has a right to dispose as she wishes of that "piece of tissue" which contains the seed of a full grown person, we shall plummet ever faster towards a brave new world in which the only barrier to the manipulation of fellow human beings will be lack of power and technique.

Opponents of abortion fear that the inhabitants of the brave new world will be possessed and driven by a type of character that will brook no interference with their ambitions from nature, man, or God. If the dystopia they envision were a certain consequence of present toleration of abortion, many moderates might reconsider their mild reformist views. But the consequences are not inevitable nor would they be horrifying to all. In light of the broad and intense demand for abortion, can the state withhold permission solely on the basis of speculation about the possible effects of abortion upon individual character?

The argument that "easy abortion" will undermine a quality of individual character necessary to uphold civic virtue suffices only to gain a place for abortion within the category of "crimes without victims." In that category, antiabortion legislation maintains a perennially perilous existence in company with laws against drug addiction, homosexuality, prostitution, and gambling. The paternalistic style of such laws is deemed old fashioned by many citizens who are only slightly to the left of the center of the spectrum. In their minds, what a man chooses to do to his individual character ought to be considered a private affair. If there is to be a justification of antiabortion legislation grounded firmly in the defense of the public interest, the search must go on.

THE POPULATION ARGUMENT: A BOOMERANG

One attempt to ground antiabortion laws in concern for the common public interest of the secular state has backfired. Throughout most of the last hundred years the strong antagonism of the churches to abortion abetted the population policies of Western nations which aimed at increasing the birth rate in order to counter the threat of underpopulation. There was a convenient alliance of secular nationalism and ecclesiastical natalism. The moral evil of abortion was also a social evil which would deny the state a citizen, a soldier, a producer. Homilies on family life frequently placed strong emphasis upon the obligation of the Christian couple, when contemplating the number of children to be brought into the world, to consider the needs of the state.

Now the demographic situation has changed. Overpopulation rather than underpopulation is a menace. The argument that couples should consider the needs of the state in deciding about their procreative behavior can prove embarrassing when public policy seeks a reduction of the birth rate. The recent demographic history of Japan is cited by many demographers as evidence that the provision of cheap and easy abortion is the most effective means of bringing about a rapid decline in the birth rate. In certain circumstances the public interest might, therefore, require the promotion rather than the discouragement of abortion.

The response of the right wing has been to deemphasize the Christian's obligation to weigh the current demographic needs of the state as a significant factor in decisions regarding family size. Instead, much labor has been expended upon the construction of a high wall of privacy which would shelter decisions regarding procreation from the influence or intervention of any public authority. Here the right wing concurs with the left. In certain contexts the Roman Catholic Bishops of the United States have expressed great deference for the principle of self-determination and the right of privacy, values central to their protagonists in the abortion debate. They invoked, for instance, "the inviolability of the right of human privacy" and "the freedom of spouses to determine the size of their families" to argue that states must abstain from exerting pressure upon the poor to practice birth control [26]. In language reminiscent of civil libertarians on the left wing of the spectrum, the Bishops have "warned of the dangers to the right of privacy." In the abortion debate, the two extreme positions seem to agree that public authority must not tamper with decisions regarding procreation.

A decision to have an abortion is viewed on the left wing simply as a particular kind of "decision regarding procreation." It falls within the sphere of private acts sheltered from public interference. As a necessary backstop to fallible contraceptive measures, abortion is indispensable to the full realization of self-determination. On the right wing, however, abortion is categorized differently. It is a decision regarding procreation, but it can never be merely private because the taking of a life is entailed. The taking of life is always a matter of public concern. It is quite properly a matter of legal restriction. This is the ground upon which antiabortion laws must rest. It is a matter of common justice and not merely of uncommon charity.

ABORTION AS A VIOLATION OF "THE RIGHT TO LIFE"

Opponents of abortion labor under the handicap of attempting to portray subtle harms to remote subjects. They find it difficult to offset the vividness of the case for abortion which can be presented on behalf of a forlorn woman whose plight can readily be discerned. There is one type of injury, however, that is vivid and is clearly within the duty of the state to prevent: murder. Right-wing authors habitually assimilate the destruction of life in abortion to the forensic category of murder. Abortion is held to violate a legally enforceable "right to life." A simple syllogism unfolds into a complex network of ideas. Human life is not to be destroyed; fetal life is human life; therefore, fetal life is not to be destroyed.

Resort to the legal vocabulary to capture the emotionally powerful term "murder" imposes an obligation to attain the linguistic precision appropriate to the legal sphere. Hence, the meaning of the major and the minor premises and the conclusion itself must be specified more closely.

The major premise represents a restriction of responsibility to protect life within confines more narrow than those implied by such terms as "reverence for life" or "respect for life." Not all life is included in the injunction, only human life. But, it is noted, even with regard to human life, the framers of the syllogism do permit exceptions. In imposing capital punishment, for example, society demands the life of one who, by his depradations upon his fellow men, is said to have forfeited his right to life. Thus the premise must be narrowed: *Innocent* human life is not to be destroyed. Again there are exceptions. In wartime, men acting in good conscience under the principle of double effect, may destroy the life of a civilian who, innocent both subjectively and materially, is tragically situated close to an important military target. A further specification is required: *Innocent* human life is not to be destroyed *by direct, purposeful attack.*

The minor premise requires not refinement but evidence of its truth in fact. Robert Drinan, S.J., Dean of Boston College Law School, has asserted, "If the advocates of legalized abortion desire to have an intellectually honest debate about the fundamental change they seek in the moral and legal standards of American life, they should not fall back on the error of fact that a fetus is not a human being" [13:123]. What type of fact is it that a fetus is a human being? What evidence would count for or against such an assertion? What type of question is posed when one asks, "Is the fetus a human being?"

In the present context, the question is, in the first instance, a legal inquiry. It translates into the question, "Can a fetus be the victim of murder?" Murder requires a human victim. Even if the fetus is not taken to be *fully* human, a moral problem still exists. One can still ask whether or not it is right to destroy whatever it is that exists in the womb after conception and before birth. Arguments against such destruction can be given which do not hinge on the question whether murder has been committed upon a fully human fetus. If the fetus is not human, what is lost is not the moral quandary regarding abortion but the strong argument for public legislation grounded in the demands of justice. If there is no human victim to be murdered, opponents of abortion must revert to less stirring arguments.

How might one "prove" the statement that "the fetus is fully human"? In order to gain the semblance of certainty over against the seemingly arbitrary demonstration available through legal or moral discourse, many right-wing authors attempt to convert the question of when human life exists into a straightforward biological problem. The question is presumed to fall within the specialty of embryology. Eugene Quay has written:

> The Christian position against the destruction of human life before or after birth never changed, but biological thought did. . . . The development of a code of law for the Church's

own governance required definition and distinction. When are we dealing with a human life?

The answer had to be found not in moral theology or ethics but in embryology [31:426].

Such an attempt to surround a moral and legal judgment with an aura of biological factuality evades the truth that, in searching for signs of life, the biologist who does not aspire himself to be a theologian must rely upon the indices of life which the theologian has defined. If the theologian says that the drawing of breath is the sign of life, the biologist is likely to report that life is not present until a moment after birth. If human life is thought to begin when a human form is visually recognizable, the biologist must estimate the moment in gestation at which the fetus becomes so "formed." If life is defined in terms of the capacity to carry on certain biological functions, it is nevertheless the theologian who has determined that these shall serve as the appropriate criteria of life.

Nor can certainty about the fully human status of the fetus be gained by recourse to philosophical and religious thought about the soul as the animating principle or actuating cause of individual life. The question then becomes even less credibly an issue to be settled by embryologists. How would their scientific tools detect the creative act of God at the moment he animates the fetus with a living soul? Theologians again must be summoned to describe what to look for. But they have disagreed among themselves. In the last hundred years, authoritative Roman Catholic teaching has required the assumption that animation takes place at the moment of conception. But many respectable theologians, past and present, have held theories of successive animation according to which the soul develops gradually through vegetative and animal stages before the distinctively human rational soul appears. Moral theologians have disagreed precisely because there is no conclusive evidence to be brought to bear from biology or from any other discipline outside of their own field. They can neither escape the decision nor invest it with a factitious certainty. In determining what it is that is to be protected through restrictions upon abortion they define what is to be considered "human life."

To pose the questions "What is human life?" and "When does human life begin?" in the midst of the abortion debate is a roundabout way of asking whether it is morally and legally permissible to destroy the matter in the womb of a pregnant woman. The reason for taking the roundabout way is to pick up en route the emotionally powerful terms "human life" and "murder" which are necessary to an argument which draws its impact from the implication, "You and your loved ones may be next if the restraints upon the taking of life are eroded at this point." The insistence upon the continuity between fetal life and adult life makes more credible the prediction of a continuity of effect from the sacrifice of the unborn child to the murder of adults.

In discussing the question, "When does human life begin?" Glanville Williams, a prominent British advocate of abortion law reform, Professor of English Law at Cambridge University and President of the Abortion Law Reform Association in England observes, "The line is one we have to draw for ourselves. And, in the absence of divine revelation, might we not allow ourselves to draw it at a point that is humanly convenient" [40:18; 41]? The point is well taken. The abortion debate is concerned with the question, "What is humanly convenient?" Christian opponents of abortion have, in fact, drawn the line which defines when human life is present at the point calculated to provide maximum support for their argument that, from the moment of conception, the fetus is fully human; destruction of its life is, therefore, murder; and condonation of murder is not humanly convenient.

The disadvantage of this argument is that it involves a considerable straining for effect. In search of rhetorical power, right-wing publicists tend to disregard pertinent distinctions which have led to the discrimination in popular language and law between "murder" and "abortion." The lack of disciplined precision invites a counterindulgence by left-wing authors. The straining for effect is aggravated when the right wing claim that the fetus is truly human is logically extended and emotionally undergirded with a religious appeal that prospective "murderers" have concern for the eternal destiny of the soul of the fetus. The fragile fabric of argument begins to tear when stretched so far. Neither the church nor the state nor the family actually carries out the practices logically entailed by the affirmation that the fetus is fully human. The church does not baptize the outpouring spontaneously aborted soon after conception. Extreme unction is not given. Funeral rites are not performed. The state calculates age from the date of birth, not of conception, and does not require a death or burial certificate nor even a report of the demise of a fetus aborted early in pregnancy. Convicted abortionists are not subjected to the penalties for murder. The intensity of grief felt within a family over a miscarriage is typically less than that experienced upon the loss of an infant, an older child, or an adult.

It is not the fate of the fetus itself that is the troubling aspect of abortion. It is difficult for most people to imagine the fetus "suffering" either here or hereafter. Indeed, much of its vulnerability stems from men's inability to believe that the fetus has a self-conscious awareness of its own existence and prospective nonexistence. The moral outrage and fear in expectation of death ascribed to a more mature victim stirs a sense of identification which few can feel with a tiny embryo.

Glanville Williams inadvertently provides a clue to the basis of the moral condemnation of abortion: "Our comparative indifference towards the natural death of the foetus contrasts strangely with the emotions traditionally released by its artificial termination" [42:61]. The significant distinction between spontaneous miscarriage and induced abortion is that the artificial termination of pregnancy involves the intervention of human agency. The natural death of the fetus is a natural evil. Induced abortion is a moral evil. It is the doing of evil, not the experiencing of evil, that is to be condemned. It is the effect that abortion is presumed to have upon the killers rather than upon the killed that makes abortion dreadful.

But if the fetus is not harmed, how can abortion be harmful? If no identifiable subject is injured by an act, how can that act be considered evil? Perhaps the concept of "harm" has again been too crude. Legal terminology provides a means of expressing a more subtle harm, a harm inflicted by the negation of the unborn child's "right to life." Every human being, by virtue of his existence, may be invested with a natural "right to life." But in order to surround the fetus with the moral immunity from direct attack to which the possession of the "right to life" entitles him, it is necessary to assume that the fetus is human. Legal concepts such as "the right to life" and "murder" can help to dramatize the implications of the affirmation that the fetus is fully human, but they cannot establish the basic point itself, which remains a matter for affirmation rather than demonstration.

The inescapable difficulty, obscured but not erased by an overlay of biological, theological, and legal suppositions, is that many people do not consider the fetus to be fully human and there is no way that they can be logically compelled so to believe. There are undeniable differences between the nonviable fetus and the fully human adult or even the newly born infant. The nonviable fetus is physically bound to its mother and may constitute a threat to her life. It is unable to be adopted or removed to the care of another. It is totally dependent upon the mother. No other arrangement can be made for its continued life. If it should become possible through transplanting the fetus to insure its continued life and development apart from the woman who conceived it, the moral problem of abortion would be changed but not abolished. Arguments which assimilate abortion to murder would be ineffective, but the claim that, for the sake of character, women should bear responsibility for nurturing that which they have conceived might still be urged.

It is inappropriate for adherents of the right wing to deny that these basic facts are devoid of significance in reasoning about abortion. But it is equally inappropriate for those on the left wing to deny that even the newest conceptus is something more than "just another piece of the woman's tissue." It is a potential man. Abortion is not just another surgical procedure. Nor is it murder. Abortion is abortion. It is a peculiar moral problem that can neither be "solved" by clumsy analogies nor dissolved by some rhetorical sleight of hand. Abortion is the destruction of potential, potential which has already attained the form of nascent life. The rejection of abortion implies an affirmation of the goodness of creation. It gives testimony to the conviction that what is potential ought to be welcomed to actuality.

It can be replied that no one except a dyspeptic nihilist would argue that abortion is good because the destruction of life is desirable in itself. The claim of reformers is only that under extraordinary circumstances abortion may be justifiable as the lesser evil. The unknown potential of the fetus must be weighed against the actualized relationships and responsibilities of the mother. The mother, as well as her unborn child, has unrealized potential. When the balance between them must be struck how should the scales be weighted?

ASSESSING THE "VALUE" OF LIFE

Those who would indulge in such calculations can employ one of two patterns of reasoning. They may give weight to the very existence of actualized potential or to the anticipated quality of unactualized potential. The first approach could be described as the "labor theory of value." Garrett Hardin expresses an attitude that inevitably leads to preference for the mother: "The early stages of an individual fetus have had very little human effort invested in them; they are of very little worth" [20:4]. A kindred view has been baptized by a clerical spokesman for the British Abortion Law Reform Association:

> Always the interests of that which is developed and formed, i.e. the mother, must take precedence over the interests of that which is embryonic and unformed, for *in the eyes of God* it is surely the living person who is all important — that separate and independent whole, identifiable as such, who at the moment of *birth* begins that process of personality development which does not cease with the cessation of life here but continues in "other mansions" of the universe [1:4; italics added].

This is a curious anthropomorphic projection onto God of the difficulties finite utilitarians encounter in decision making. It is understandable that some men, bound to a tiny span of time and thus unable to predict the future of the fetus, might prefer the assessible if modest "worth" of the mother. But, if God is a utilitarian, he has the advantage of being an omniscient utilitarian. The eyes of God might foresee that certain unborn children would achieve inestimably more than the mothers intent upon aborting them. If his intention were to preserve the life that might, through a large span of time, bring the greatest good to the greatest number, preference could not automatically be given to that which at one moment happens to be more fully developed and formed. The choice of the mother is at best a tragic risk imposed by human finitude; it is foolish to bless it as a faithful and certain imitation of what God would do.

As men become more godlike in the scope if not in the employment of their powers, surprising conclusions may be drawn by application of a second mode of reasoning which, in emphasizing the quality of unrealized potential, need not lead to the automatic preference of the mother over her unborn child. By shifting the unknowables in a not uncommon decision-making formula we may perform a thought experiment which, if medically improbable, is nevertheless ethically interesting. Suppose a situation late in pregnancy where it is medically possible to save either but not both the mother and child. Suppose, further, that the state of fetology has advanced so that it can be predicted confidently that the offspring will be of very superior endowment. The mother is, by universal agreement, a wretch. Considering the potential benefit to the community and the quality of individual life that could be attained, would it not be deemed suitable to kill the mother in order to insure the realization of the superior potential of her child?

This second mode of reasoning should appeal to social engineers imbued with a perfectionist streak. It would enhance their opportunities to assist in the process of the natural selection of the fittest and thus accelerate the "improvement of the race." Indeed, it might come to be considered an indispensable argument for the legitimation of "racial self-determination" if such a concept were to be challenged on behalf of the unfit and unwanted as a menace to their right of individual self-determination.

Concern for the "quality of life" or "the full realization of human potential" can be used well to stimulate efforts to prevent the occurrence of lamentable defects and deficiencies so that all may enjoy a high quality of life. But it can also lead to an inclination to derogate life which, burdened with defects and deficiencies, does not seem capable of high quality. The application of "quality control" techniques to the production of new life is a constant temptation to some. An ominous note is sounded in an article by a Protestant layman and physician Dr. H. B. Munson, who writes, "these days it seems a questionable practice even to allow an irresponsible mother to take responsibility for the rearing of a child, much less force her to do so. . . . The fact that these days we not only allow her to keep her baby, but that to a large degree we force this state of affairs by denying her an abortion would seem to make us guilty of mismanagement" [25:9]. Dr. Munson, seems to be on the verge of proposing an indication for *involuntary* abortion which would be imposed for the sake of maintaining a well managed society. One cannot repress the question, "Who will be the managers?"

It is important that the question concerning the nature of true "quality" be pressed continually. Christians, secular humanists, and other men of good will may jointly insist that the very definition of "quality of life" must include toleration, respect, and active concern for those who are aged, weak, deformed, unskilled, cantankerous, or perverse. If we are to be civilized at all, those who attain true "quality of life" must exhibit a spirit of *noblesse oblige*. (Christian theologians may properly complain that the concept of "noblesse oblige" does not do justice to the radical quality of *agape* held up for emulation in the Gospel. Those who aspire to live and die by the norm of Christian charity may be called to exhibit a higher "quality of life" in yielding convenience, health, or life itself in self-sacrificing concern to preserve the life of the fetus, just as God in Christ gave up that which was most precious to give true life to those of little worth.)

It seems there are few who are able to sustain the theological beliefs necessary to give meaning to the realization of potential through self-sacrifice for the sake of the life of another. But Americans habitually do glorify the sacrifice of life in defense of the nation. And heroes frequently risk and not infrequently lose their lives in the rescue of fellow men. Yet the sacrifice of a mother to save the unknown, nascent, potential life contained in a tiny tissue is not heralded on civic occasions. It is the apparent disproportion of the sacrifice that seems objectionable. The more the life of the fetus is depreciated, the more glaring is the apparent disproportion. Dr. Munson states, "After all, one can hardly equate, on the one hand, the taking of life from a breathing, thinking, full-fledged human being, with, on the other hand, the denial of life to a bit of vegetating unborn matter, that, so far as we can tell, is unable to suffer and apparently doesn't even have any awareness of its own existence" [25:9].

Behind this reaction is "the labor theory of value" which suggests that it is man's labor, his hopes and purposes, his investment of financial aid and psychological capital which bestows a value upon human life. The "worth" of a life grows as its place within the consciousness of others expands. The degree of protection to be afforded the fetus increases as it becomes more and more a focal point of others' dreams and plans. That which defines fully human existence is the capacity for social interaction which brings forth the ultimate value of "human personality." Many persons have poured their labor into the formation of the personality of a mother. To exchange that realized potential for the uncertain future of an unresponsive entity incapable of self-conscious intercourse with human beings would be to squander a scarce resource. It would be an uneconomic transaction.

This style of reasoning could leave every man uncertain whether he had attained "fully human" status. It would give little moral protection to those who might be stunted in their social development, less to the comatose, and none to the moribund.

The significance of defining "fully human existence" in terms of capacity for self-conscious social interaction is suggested in a passage from a pamphlet issued by the Board of Social Ministry of the Lutheran Church in America:

> Furthermore, in Christian decision-making, while one must regard incipient human life as precious, he will have to distinguish between its claims and those of more developed human life. The fetus or newborn infant that has been called into human existence by God's address bears in a formal sense the image of God, stands in enduring relationship to Him, and has the extremely valuable potential for a loving human response to God and other human beings. Yet there is a qualitative difference between such a being and the mature person who is a free center of decision and responsibility, with a history and present capacity for full-blown, loving relationships with other persons.

The "qualitative difference between such a being and a mature person" opens the way for the authors to recommend "compassionate abortion" for medical, psychiatric, eugenic, humanitarian, and socioeconomic reasons. Their "proposed strategy comes close to recent Scandinavian practice." It is intended not simply as a reluctant concession in public law to nonbelievers but as a guide to the "decisional life of the Christian woman considering abortion" [39:15, 25, 19].

Both the emphasis of "the labor theory of value" upon the degree of realized human potential, and the social engineering stress upon the quality of unrealized potential represent departures from the classical Christian account of the origin of the worth of each human life. Christians have proclaimed that God has bestowed upon man "an alien dignity" [38:231]. Man's worth is not to be assessed according to what he has become through social intercourse or by an estimate of what he may yet become. Rather, it is God's labor, his purpose, his economy which places the price of each life so high that no transient human value can serve as compensation. But, with the erosion of the theological foundations of the Christian view of man's alien dignity, the barriers to abortion built upon those foundations are crumbling in the hearts of individuals and in the statutes of the states. The

trend may be lamentable, but the demands of Christian responsibility cannot be met by pouting and pining for a "age of faith."
What must the churches do now in the face of a problem they
will no longer be allowed to ignore?

OPTIONS FOR THE CHURCHES

The drift of the abortion debate is clearly to the left. An ironic
benefit of the confusion which has beset the Protestant churches
is that it has kept open several options. Different streams might
be panned in the search for a new wealth of ideas.

The new receptivity of Protestants to arguments for abortion
law reform has been attributed to a decline of the theological
certainties which supported right-wing arguments; to the ex-
ploitation of latent Protestant themes to bolster the left-wing demand for self-determination and control over nature, including
human nature; and to perplexity concerning the proper relationship between the moral beliefs of particular segments of the public and legal enactments imposed upon all of the citizenry.
Alternative strategies might emerge through response to one or
another of these factors.

One possibility is to attempt to reverse the tide and rebuild the
eroded theological foundations of the ban on abortion so that narrow restraints might be enforced both within the church and
within society. A second course is to proceed to the blessing and
baptizing of the arguments of the left wing and a willing entry
into a brave new world in the hope that churchmen, having supplied some of the building materials, might have a role in shaping
the plan of the new city of man. A third option is to accede to
the separation of the legal and the moral and withdraw into a sectarian absolutism, preserving the ban on abortion under the
discipline of the church but relinquishing the determination of
public policy to other voices.

Each of these three options has disadvantages. The first requires confidence in the possibility of theological reconstruction

and the renewal of profound religious commitment throughout a broad segment of the American public. Even many who pray for such a revival would be startled by its occurrence. The second option entails a theological reconstitution involving the abandonment of significant elements of Christian teaching about the nature of human life and the obligation to preserve it. The discontinuity would be jarring to the churches. The changes would ramify throughout the entire system of Christian doctrine. Teaching upon related social and moral issues would have to be recast. The implications for Christian thought concerning the obligation to show respect for life in other settings might be unappealing even, or perhaps, especially to those who now advocate accommodation of Christians to the idea of abortion on demand. The third approach implies a sociological reformation of the relationship of the churches to matters of public policy in a variety of fields. If the churches withdraw from the struggle on behalf of the fetus to defend by law the most fundamental "right to life" how will they be brought back into the public arena to do battle on behalf of the rights of racial minorities, the poor, the persecuted, the victims of injustice and warfare? Whatever measure of grace, love, and justice the churches are able to mediate needs to be diffused throughout the public realm and not be confined within a sectarian enclave. It would be a bad bargain for all if the cost of removing "obstinate" churchmen from the abortion controversy were to be the diminution of their active public concern for abolition of poverty and the realization of civil rights, peace, and a more just world order.

A fourth option constitutes the most probable outcome of the churches' increasing concern with the problem of abortion. The mainline Protestant churches can be expected to provide spotty support for reform measures modeled on the American Law Institute proposals. It is doubtful that abortion law reform will become a cause promoted by a fervent Protestant crusade. But when the issue is thrust upon them, Protestants will respond with an uncoordinated but steady movement toward acceptance of moderate reform. When statewide controversies reach a critical stage in which debate is polarized between Roman Catholic spokesmen in the right wing and advocates of abortion on demand on the left, Protestants will gravitate toward the middle. They will be moved by political disposition rather than by theological exposition. After their arrival, they will need to fill in theological ground on which to stand.

To date, there has been little progress in the endeavor to shore up the position towards which Protestants seem to be edging. Extended battles over abortion law reform in New York and California have brought forth outpourings of polemic utterances. But no substantial, original study of the theological and ethical dimensions of the abortion issue has been produced by American Protestant churchmen. Readers have been forced to rely upon materials translated from German or imported from England [38; 5; 4; 7].

By the time American Protestants are prepared to address the issue of abortion in its present manifestations it is likely that new developments will have recast the current questions. The development of an abortifacient pill that might be prescribed for simple, private, inexpensive, safe use at home will alter the pattern of debate over abortion. Issues that hinge upon estimates of effects of illegal abortion upon mothers, the medical profession, law enforcement agencies, and the poor will become less salient, as will controversies regarding the utility of procedural devices such as hospital abortion committees. A new phase of debate will evolve, a phase in which polarization will be increased. Self-determination will seem to be more readily within reach. Women could abort without risky dependence upon a shady underworld and without the reallocation of scarce medical resources necessary to provide abortion on demand under present medical conditions. But the violation of the "right to life" of the fetus will be the same.

Unless the abortifacient pill is made available to all women, married and unmarried, in all circumstances, new problems of control will arise and a new debate regarding "contraindications" will evolve. It will still be necessary to balance contending values that appear to be both indispensable and incompatible. The immediate terms of debate may change. But the need for precise ethical analysis of fundamental issues will not change. Even if the tiniest sliver of life can be extinguished quietly at home by a mother uncertain of its existence, abortion will continue to be a problem worthy of Christian concern.

CAN THE DEMAND FOR ABORTION BE REDUCED?

The prospect of a safe abortifacient pill available for self-administration at home quickens awareness of the inefficacy of all external sanctions against abortion. If the demand for abortion were high, effective suppression of the pill would be difficult to achieve. But even today, when most abortions require clandestine negotiations and a costly surgical procedure, those who seek to reduce the number of abortions cannot expect success merely through more aggressive enforcement of criminal provisions or the imposition of more strict administrative procedures in hospitals. They must seek to allay the demand for abortion through a variety of social innovations which might increase a pregnant woman's inclination to bear her child by (1) easing the burden of pregnancy through the provision of better medical care and opportunities for consultation, improvement in the status of illegitimate children, and greater tolerance of unwed mothers; (2) providing assurance of proper care for the child, either *apart* from the mother, through more adequate programs for foster homes and adoption, or *with* the mother through alleviation of poverty by improved programs of social welfare, family subsidy, or tax relief, and through the creation of day-care facilities. The most popular approach to the reduction of the demand for abortion is to reduce unwanted pregnancies through better sex education and the promotion of improved contraceptive practices.

The possible effectiveness of contraception as a means of forestalling the desire for abortion has been used within the Roman Catholic Church as an argument on behalf of a more liberal attitude toward birth control programs. But many Roman Catholic commentators agree with advocates of abortion on demand that contraception and abortion will inevitably be linked in practice. Both extremes consider the hope of having one without the other to be chimeric. Believers in justifiable abortion find consolation in the anticipation that more aggressive promotion of contraception will diminish the demand for abortion by preventing unwanted pregnancies.

But the extreme schools join in the observation that, in order to motivate couples to use contraceptives, it is necessary to generate a strong intention not to have another child at a particular moment in time. By inducing this strong motivation, one simultaneously stimulates a latent demand for abortion should contraception fail. Advocates of abortion on demand conclude that "Abortion is the much-needed backstop in the system of birth control" [19:80]. Right-wing authors predict that once a "contraceptive mentality" has been cultivated and interference with the lifegiving process has been permitted a slide downward toward "murder for convenience" is inevitable.

It is all but impossible not to feel that one has been cheated when an unexpected pregnancy arrives in spite of the prophylactic methods authorized by law. One naturally turns to the legislator who is indirectly guilty of having approved an imperfect and defective technique whose results are unexpected and disappointing. He must be asked to supplement such dubious legislation by allowing abortion to those whose belief in the effectiveness of a contraceptive technique has proved unfounded.

In fact, this is precisely what we see happening in countries which have legalized contraception. Their legislation inevitably leads the way to so-called therapeutic, eugenic and social laws whose purpose it is to correct the errors and deficiencies of the prophylactic measures [24:56].

It is not unreasonable to conclude that the high demand for abortion is stimulated not exclusively by social ills but by a disposition of the spirit of the age. The clientele of criminal abortionists includes the poor and the unmarried, but it consists primarily of married women, comfortably placed, who bear neither shame nor poverty, but are resolved to preserve or extend whatever comfort they have attained. No program or policy readily at the disposal of the public can quickly change the calculations that lead women to conclude that abortion is the most convenient solution to their awkward, but not tragic, circumstance.

Abortion can be seen as a medical, legal, social, and ethical problem. It also is to be seen as a problem involving the meaning of life. No external authority can reimpose respect for the law regulating abortion. Apart from such respect, the social costs of enforcement become exorbitant. If legal restraints are to function they must be buttressed by inner conviction. But the conviction has decayed that abortion is an offense against God, nature, the state, one's higher self, the common weal, and the right to life. Can it ever flourish again?

Those who, for one reason or another, would like to reduce the incidence of abortion, must ask, "How can 'respect for life' be regenerated?" The famous Swiss Protestant theologian, Karl Barth, believes that in all but the extraordinary case in which life is pitted against life, the church must continue to urge the state to say "No" to abortion.

> The question arises, however, how this "No" is to be established and stated if it is to be a truly effective "No." In the face of the wicked violation of the sanctity of life which is always seriously at issue in abortion, and which is always present when it is carried out thoughtlessly and callously, the only thing which can help is the power wholly new and radical feeling of awe at the mystery of all human life as this is commanded by God as its Creator, Giver and Lord. Legal prohibitions and restrictions of a civil, moral and supposedly spiritual kind are obviously inadequate to instill this awe into man. Nor does mere churchmanship, whether Romanist or Protestant, provide the atmosphere in which this awe can thrive [4:417 f].

This reminder can bring both chagrin and challenge to the churches. The radical feeling of awe at the mystery of all human life can never be predictably induced. But it is best conveyed by demonstrating respect for life in all its forms through the courage of an institution or an individual to sacrifice wealth and prestige and station in defense of the poor, the sick, the homeless, the confused, the aged, the outcast in the ghetto, and the victims of war. Selective and painless opposition to evil is not impressive. The day of renewed inner restraints upon abortion will come sooner if churchmen and theologians exhibit in their relations with all men the same sacrifice of self in love which they have required of mothers menaced by their own offspring. A fetus may deserve respect because it is no less precious than a man. But neither should a man be less the object of ecclesiastical concern than a fetus. The churches must bridge their own credibility gap with costly grace, if they wish others to attain the grace to see the cost of each abortion.

The "cure" of the abortion epidemic can be no less profound than its causes. If, as right-wing critics affirm, its source is in the heart of man, its remedy must penetrate to similar depths. Neither cool debate nor heated polemics can move men at such levels. Only the example of sincere regard for others can rekindle the conviction that all life is sacred and bound together in mystery so that the death of the least diminishes each.

When a fetus is aborted no one asks for whom the bell tolls. No bell is tolled. But do not feel indifferent and secure. The fetus symbolizes you and me and our tenuous hold upon a future here at the mercy of our fellow men.

REFERENCES

1. The Abortion Law Reform Association: A Clergyman's View (pamphlet, London, England) no date, p 4.
2. American Law Institute Model Penal Code, Section 230.3 (proposed official draft) 1962.
3. American Lutheran Church: *Responsible Reproduction* (Commission on Research and Social Action, The American Lutheran Church, Minneapolis, Minnesota) 1967, paragraph 17, p 6.
4. Barth, Karl: *Church Dogmatics: The Doctrine of Creation,*

III, 4 (T & T Clark, Edinburgh, Scotland) 1961, pp 415 – 422; 417 f.

5. Bonhoeffer, Dietrich: *Ethics*, Eberhard Bethge, ed (SCM Press, London, England) 1960, pp 130–131.

6. Calderone, Mary S, ed: Report of the Statistics Committee, *Abortion in the United States: A Conference Sponsored by the Planned Parenthood Federation of America, Inc, at Arden House and the New York Academy of Medicine* (Hoeber Division, Harper and Row, Publishers, New York, New York) 1958, pp 57, 180.

7. Church Assembly Board for Social Responsibility: *Abortion: An Ethical Discussion* (Church Assembly Board for Social Responsibility, London, England) 1965, the most substantial theological and ethical analysis of abortion to be produced by a Protestant body in English-speaking nations.

8. Devereux, George: A Typological Study of Abortion in 350 Primitive, Ancient, and Pre-Industrial Societies, in Harold Rosen, ed: *Therapeutic Abortion: Medical, Psychiatric, Legal, Anthropological and Religious Considerations* (The Julian Press, New York, New York) 1954, pp 97–152.

9. Devereux, George: *A Study of Abortion in Primitive Societies* (The Julian Press, New York, New York) 1955.

10. Diocese of California: *The Pacific Churchman*, vol 98, no 4, Apr 1967.

11. Diocese of Central New York: *Abortion: a Position Paper, Adopted June 8, 1967, by the Council of the Episcopal Diocese of Central New York and Commended to Parish Groups and Vestries for Study* (Diocese of Central New York, Syracuse, New York) 1967.

12. Drinan, Robert F, S.J.: Strategy on Abortion, *America*, Feb 4, 1967, pp 177–179.

13. Drinan, Robert F, S.J.: The Inviolability of the Right to Be Born, *Abortion and the Law*, in David T Smith, ed (Western Reserve University Press, Cleveland, Ohio) 1967, p 123.

14. Fletcher, Joseph: A Moral Tension and an Ethical Frontier, *The Christian Scholar*, vol 46, no 3, Fall 1963, p 261.

15. Fletcher, Joseph: *Situation Ethics* (Westminster Press, Philadelphia, Pennsylvania) 1966.

16. Gebhard, Paul H; Pomeroy, Wardell B; Martin, Clyde E; and Christenson, Cornelia V: *Pregnancy, Birth and Abortion* (Harper and Row, Publishers, New York, New York) 1958, pp 197 f.

17. George, B James, jr: Current Abortion Laws: Proposals and Movements for Reform, in David T Smith, ed: *Abortion and the Law* (Western Reserve University Press, Cleveland, Ohio) 1967, pp 1–36, helpful analysis of legal materials.

18. Guttmacher, Alan F, ed: *The Case for Legalized Abortion Now* (Diablo Press, Berkeley, California) 1967, the most extensive compendium of contemporary left-wing essays.

19. Hardin, Garrett: Abortion and Human Dignity, in Alan F Guttmacher, ed: *The Case for Legalized Abortion Now* (Diablo Press, Berkeley, California) 1967, p 75.

20. Hardin, Garrett: A Scientist's Case for Abortion, reprinted from *Redbook*, May 1967, by the Association for the Study of Abortion, p 4.

21. Kinsolving, Lester: What About Therapeutic Abortion? *The Christian Century*, vol 81, no 20, May 13, 1964, pp 632–635.

22. Kummer, Jerome M, and Leavy, Zad: Therapeutic Abortion Law Confusion, *The Journal of the American Medical Association*, vol 195, no 2, Jan 10, 1966, p 97.

23. Lehmann, Paul L: *Ethics in a Christian Context* (Harper and Row, Publishers, New York, New York) 1963, p 54.

24. Lestapis, Stanislas de, S.J.: *Family Planning and Modern Problems: A Catholic Analysis* (Herder and Herder, New York, New York) 1961, chap 7, Contraceptive Civilization.

25. Munson, H B: Abortion in Modern Times: Thoughts and Comments, *The South Dakota Journal of Medicine*, vol 19, Apr 1966, pp 23–30, republished in *Renewal*, Feb 1967, p 9.

26. National Catholic Welfare Conference: Statement issued by the Administrative Board of the National Catholic Welfare Conference, Washington, D.C., Nov 14, 1966, in *The Boston Pilot*, Nov 19, 1966.

27. National Council of the Churches of Christ: *Responsible Parenthood: A Pronouncement Adopted by the General*

Board, Feb 23, 1961 (National Council of the Churches of Christ, New York, New York) 1961, p 2.

28. The National Council of the Episcopal Church: *The Family Today: The Report of Committee Five of the Lambeth Conference, 1958* (The National Council of the Episcopal Church, New York, New York) no date, p 15.

29. Pilpel, Harriet: The Abortion Crisis, in Alan F Guttmacher, ed: *The Case for Legalized Abortion Now* (Diablo Press, Berkeley, California) 1967, especially p 113.

30. Quay, Eugene: Justifiable Abortion: Medical and Legal Foundations, *The Georgetown Law Journal*, vol 49, no 2, Winter 1960, pp 173–256, see also reference 31.

31. Quay, Eugene: Justifiable Abortion: Medical and Legal Foundations, *The Georgetown Law Journal*, vol 49, no 3, Spring 1961, pp 395–538. An extensive bibliography accompanies the article, the first portion of which is in reference 30. A 73-page summary of laws governing abortion in the United States and its territories is contained in an appendix.

32. Ramsey, Paul: The Case of Joseph Fletcher and Joseph Fletcher's Cases, in *Deeds and Rules in Christian Ethics* (Charles Scribner's Sons, New York, New York) 1967, p 168; for Ramsey's views on abortion, see The Sanctity of Life: In the First of It, *The Dublin Review*, Spring 1967.

33. Rossi, Alice S: Public Views on Abortion, unpublished report of the National Opinion Research Center, Feb 1966. The paper is now available in Alan F Guttmacher, ed: *The Case for Legalized Abortion Now* (Diablo Press, Berkeley, California) 1967, pp 26–53. See also Abortion Laws and Their Victims, *Trans-action* Sept–Oct 1966. The interpretation of the poll data offered here should not be ascribed to Mrs Rossi.

34. St John-Stevas, Norman: *The Right to Life* (Hodder & Stoughton, Ltd, London, England) 1963, pp 16, 17, 36, 127.

35. Schur, Edwin M: *Crimes without Victims: Deviant Behavior and Public Policy — Abortion, Homosexuality, Drug Addiction* (Prentice-Hall, Inc, Englewood Cliffs, New Jersey) 1965, pp 59, 60.

36. Society for Humane Abortion: *Statement of Policy* (pamphlet) no date.
37. Szasz, Thomas S: Bootlegging Humanistic Values through Psychiatry, *The Antioch Review*, Fall 1962, 344.
38. Thielicke, Helmut: *The Ethics of Sex*, John W Doberstein, translator (Harper and Row, Publishers, New York, New York) 1964, p 231.
39. Wentz, Frederick K, and Witmer, Robert H: *The Problem of Abortion* (Board of Social Ministry, Lutheran Church in America, New York, New York) 1967, pp 15, 25, 19.
40. Williams, Glanville: Introduction, in Alice Jenkins, *Law for the Rich* (Victor Gollancz, Ltd, London, England) 1960, p 18.
41. Williams, Glanville: *The Sanctity of Life and the Criminal Law* (Alfred A Knopf, New York, New York) 1966, one of the most extensive recent discussions of abortion in English.
42. Williams, Glanville: Moral Issues, in *Abortion in Britain: Proceedings of a Conference Held by the Family Planning Association at the University of London Union on 22 April 1966* (Pitman Medical Publishing Co, Ltd, London, England) 1966, p 61.

6. RELIGIOUS FACTORS IN THE POPULATION PROBLEM

by Arthur J. Dyck

CONCERN over what has been variously dramatized as "the population crisis," "the population dilemma," or "the population explosion" is now rather widespread. During the 1960s, mass media have liberally dispersed mounting demographic data documenting the increasingly rapid growth of world population. As Professor Roger Revelle has noted [41:2–9], it took hundreds of thousands of years to produce a living population of one billion people by 1850 A.D. Within 75 years, from 1850 to 1925, the second billion was added, and by 1960, in only 35 more years, the third billion. The world's population will exceed four billions by 1980 and five billions by 1990, a mere 10 years later. Barring considerable change in birth and death rates, the population increase between now and the year 2000 will be larger than the entire population presently living on this planet.

Beyond the relatively remote problems posed by the ultimate limits of sheer space, population growth rates in numerous areas of our globe are already outstripping existing capacities to provide the resources vital for human survival. Unfortunately, we cannot comfort ourselves with the thought that the minimal nutritional needs of such areas can, at least for some time to come, be met by contributions from societies now possessing fairly abundant food supplies. Calculations by Revelle [42:328–351] indicate that even an 80% increase in food production in the United States by 1985, no mean undertaking, would provide only 10% of what the underdeveloped world will require up to that time. Even if the rate of population growth of relatively underdeveloped areas should markedly diminish, the United States by tripling its food production could furnish less than

20% of the food needs for these areas between now and the year 2000.

These simple but sobering facts vividly pinpoint the most fundamental aspect of the population problem: the need to match population growth with food supplies. But bread alone, essential as it is, has never been seen as sufficient for the "good life." The quality of human existence is intricately tied to the quality of our total environment. Provisions for pollution abatement and for recreational, educational, aesthetic, and transportational facilities, all require some kind of rational ecological adjustment if we are to achieve more than bare subsistence on this planet or, for that matter, on any other planet.

MALTHUS' "MISERY AND VICE"

We are prone to view as strictly contemporary and unique the problems associated with the rapid growth of population. Although these problems have escalated sharply in our time, some of them are certainly not new. Scholarly reflection upon the causes and effects of population growth goes back at least as far as Malthus, whose first essay on population appeared in 1798 under the title *An Essay on the Principle of Population As It Affects the Future Improvement of Society, with Remarks on the Speculations of Mr. Godwin, Mr. Condercet, and Other Writers.* Indeed, Malthus himself, writing five years later in a revised edition of his essay, tells of the extent to which others as remote in time as Plato and Aristotle had noted "the poverty and misery arising from a too rapid increase of population"; and he expresses surprise that this subject "had not excited more of the public attention."

In the course of this inquiry I found that much more had been done than I had been aware of when I first published the Essay. The poverty and the misery arising from a too rapid increase of population had been distinctly seen, and the most violent remedies proposed so long ago as the times of Plato and Aristotle. And of late years the subject has been treated in such a manner by some French Economists, occasionally by Montesquieu, and, among our own writers, by Dr. Franklin, Sir James Steuard, Mr. Arthur Young, and Mr. Townsend, as to create a natural surprise that it had not excited more of the public attention [33:1–148].

But Malthus is aware of the shortcomings of what he had found in the literature:

> Though it had been stated distinctly, that population must always be kept down to the level of subsistence; yet few inquiries had been made into the various modes by which this level is effected; and the principle had never been sufficiently pursued to its consequences, nor had those practical inferences [been] drawn from it, which a strict examination of its effects on society appears to suggest [33:148].

Malthus, a minister in the Church of England and a professor of economics and history, is widely acknowledged as the founder or "father" of modern population study (including the science of demography). According to Thompson and Lewis, he earned this title because of his "continued and *highly objective* interest in the factors affecting population growth and in the relation between this growth and human welfare" [46:23].

Despite the rather extensive demographic research since the time of Malthus, much of it descriptive and relatively recent, we have yet to ascertain how, in a number of underdeveloped areas, it is possible to keep the level of population commensurate with the level of subsistence; and, as our earlier remarks revealed, the necessity for accomplishing this is fast becoming a worldwide, a *species* problem.

As Malthus observed, the human suffering associated with populations whose birth rates greatly exceed their death rates had been acknowledged for a long time. There have been several classical types of responses to the ills engendered by high rates of population growth, two of which were espoused by Malthus and a third by certain of his critics among the Marxists and Catholics. These classic responses interest us here because they still represent, in the most general sense, the alternatives confronting us today.

In his 1798 essay, Malthus took the view that "Misery and Vice," in the form of war, famine, disease, malnutrition, and other processes over which individual human beings have little or no control, determine the birth and death rates. For this hypothesis, precluding the possibility of preventing by human intervention the ravages of "Misery and Vice," Malthus was considered gloomy and pessimistic by his contemporaries. Although we shall not, in this essay, champion this first hypothesis of Malthus, it is important to bear in mind that no one is currently in a position to declare it patently false. We can envisage, and to some extent have actualized, ways to prevent war, famine, disease, and malnutrition; but we cannot claim that, as a species, man is clearly winning the struggle against them. There is evidence to suggest, however, that these forms of human suffering need not inevitably be engendered by overly rapid population growth, for, as Malthus observed after publishing his first essay, there are restraints operating upon birth rates which are within man's voluntary control.

MALTHUS' "MORAL RESTRAINT"

Malthus, therefore, revised his original hypothesis and proposed the following: "Moral Restraint" (plus or minus "Misery and Vice") determines the birth rate. By maintaining that birth rates are affected by deliberate human decisions and actions, and in this way kept at a comparatively low level, Malthus is allowing for the possibility of maintaining low death rates through good health practices and adequate nutrition without having, as a consequence, the sorts of growth rates that irrevocably lead to the syndrome of "Misery and Vice."

Students of population presently hold at least three compatible hypotheses of the type represented by the revised and final view taken by Malthus. All affirm the propositions that the birth rate and the death rate decrease with time and that the birth rate approaches the steady state death rate. This phenomenon, often described in demography textbooks and elsewhere as the Demographic Transition, has been the pattern observed in the Western world. The theoretical understanding of this pattern remains highly controversial and, as we shall try to show later, is critical for the success of any direct attempt to prevent rapid population growth where it is presently occurring.

The three hypotheses to which we are referring are the following: that large numbers of people feel a need to control the number of their children and will do so under the right conditions (the felt-need hypothesis); that the motivation to use Moral Restraint — that is, the desire to exercise fertility control — can be increased; and that the conditions favorable to the exercising of fertility control can be improved. We shall discuss each of these hypotheses in turn and, in the course of doing so, shall try to clarify the ways in which moral and religious variables relate to and affect fertility control.

The "right conditions" for the (felt-need) hypothesis are realized by providing reliable, relatively inexpensive, medically safe contraceptives, and advice on how to use them. The availability and distribution of both contraceptives and contraceptive information must furthermore be assured by setting up and maintaining effective administrative facilities and communication networks. In short, according to the felt-need hypothesis, birth rates will approach the steady state death rate when it is technically possible to have only the children one desires.

What evidence is there to confirm such a hypothesis? To begin with, it is clear that in most societies at most times, some men and women attempt fertility control, using a variety of means such as infanticide, abortion, prolonged breast feeding, partial or complete abstinence of sexual relations (including variants of the rhythm method), coitus interruptus and folk methods of contraception [32; 35; 24]. Furthermore, one finds that in certain of the less developed countries, most notably Taiwan, South Korea, and India, significant numbers of women have wanted to be fitted with intrauterine contraceptive devices (IUCD), and in India some men are willing to undergo vasectomy.

Indeed, these facts have been an important recent source of considerable optimism about the possibility of greatly reducing birth rates throughout the world. In one instance, Donald Bogue [8:449–454] is led to speak with transparent enthusiasm of the "demographic breakthrough" in the years 1963–1964: Such a shift from the "projection" to the "control" of fertility rates is brought about, he alleges, by a number of fertility control programs distributing contraceptives in various regions of the world, most of them in Asia in countries with very high birth rates. Bogue's declaration of a "breakthrough" at that time had to rest almost exclusively upon the fact that a fairly high proportion of the women contacted were accepting contraceptives provided by these family planning programs. In Taiwan, it is true, birth rates were noticeably declining. But there is no clear evidence that this decline in birth rates was brought about by a birth control program. Two recent surveys of family planning programs around the world by Dudley Kirk [25:48–60] and J. A. Ross [44:1–5] express a definite, though a somewhat more guarded, optimism about the prospects for the success of these programs.

Obviously, acceptance of the felt-need hypothesis directly determines the kind of strategy that is considered efficacious for bringing down birth rates; if birth rates can be sharply reduced by making efficient contraceptives and information concerning their use readily available, it is not considered essential to engage in research to find out *why* people have children and *why* they want to have a certain number. Establishing facilities and programs for effective distribution of contraceptives is believed to have virtually exclusive priority. That this belief has had considerable influence is evident from the money and effort expended by private organizations and, increasingly, by governments to establish birth control programs in "needy" areas around the world [44:1–5; 25:48–60].

Have these programs succeeded? Not one of these attempts to reduce birth rates has so far been *proved* to be instrumental. Where birth rates have declined, as in Taiwan, the decline had started before the program for contraception had been initiated, and, in the absence of controls, the cause or causes of the decline cannot unequivocally be determined. Although present efforts on behalf of fertility control represent "progress" for J. A. Ross [44], he candidly reports that "the missing link remains a proven fertility decline, resulting from deliberate effort." It is only fair to note that he is *hopeful* that such evidence will be forthcoming in two or three populations by the end of 1966. Dudley Kirk [25], surveying worldwide efforts at fertility control one year later, takes much the same view as Ross. It is noteworthy, however, that Kirk, in reporting three countries whose birth rates have declined (Taiwan, Korea, and Singapore), attributes the most marked declines in Taiwan and Korea largely to social change rather than to any past efforts directed toward family planning programs.

There is definite evidence, however, that the simple provision of advice and materials for contraception has, in certain cultures and under certain circumstances, proved futile. The very thorough research of Drs. Gordon and Wyon, conducted from 1953 – 1960 in India (the Khanna region of the Punjab) is a clear demonstration of this futility, at least for the region in question: more than half of the couples in the study accepted the advice and the contraceptives but no significant change in the birth rate resulted [50; 51]. The Lulliani study in West Pakistan, using the IUCD, obtained similar results. These findings warrant the rejection of the felt-need hypothesis as a *sufficient* account of fertility control since there are at least some populations and regions in which the behavior predicted by this hypothesis did not occur even though the conditions it posits as requisite for eliciting that behavior had been actualized.

If the felt-need hypothesis did in fact specify the necessary and sufficient conditions for bringing about birth rates that approach the steady state death rate, the moral and religious issues affecting fertility control would be relatively insignificant, limited to attitudes and doctrines regarding the use and distribution of these techniques.

FERTILITY CONTROL AND WORLD RELIGIONS

Because of its official opposition to contraceptives, the Roman Catholic Church has sometimes been singled out in the literature as the sole religious opponent of efforts to reduce birth rates throughout the world. In a survey of the demographic literature, Freedman [18] observes that many writers on underdeveloped countries stress this distinction between Catholicism and the other major religions. One might consider the Eastern Orthodox an exception here, but, as Fagley [17] has noted, their position is rather flexible.

Other major religions and religious bodies are said to form no such barrier for they do not officially condemn the use of contraceptives. Islam, in fact, has issued theologically authoritative pronouncements permitting their use under certain circumstances. In 1937, the Mufti of Egypt released a *fatwa* proclaiming, "It is permissible for either husband or wife, by mutual consent, to take any measures to prevent semen from entering the uterus, in order to prevent conception" (English translation in *Human Fertility*, vol. 10, no 2, June 1945). The *Fatwa* Committee of El Azhar University in 1953, the Directorate of Religious Affairs in Turkey in 1961, and the Grand Mufti of Jordan in 1964 also issued *fatwas* of that kind.

Thus, with premises such as these linked to the felt-need hypothesis, the *Washington Post*, for example, editorialized: "To the non-Catholic world, population control is not a religious matter; it is a quite practical matter of finding an effective means of bringing birth into harmonious relation to the ability of parents to discharge the obligation of parenthood" [28:1433]. Restricting the role of religion in this way distorts our understanding of its actual significance for the solution of the population problem. It overlooks two very important considerations: the disparity between official doctrine and actual behavior, whether this disparity is promoted by the abundance or the relative lack of some form of local piety, and the scope of moral and religious variables affecting fertility control. Failure to take the first consideration into account exaggerates the importance of Catholic doctrine and, at the same time, minimizes the importance of folk beliefs currently held within the various religious traditions. Failure to take the second consideration into account means that no recognition is made of the point at which the influence of religion upon fertility control is most decisive for the population problem.

As Ralph B. Potter has convincingly argued [38], official church doctrines in the form of papal and church pronouncements have, at best, a modest effect upon practice. One finds, for example, that the percentage of Roman Catholic women in this country complying with the Church's ban on "artificial means" of contraception declined from 70% in 1955 to 62% in 1960 and to 47% in 1965. The attitudes recently expressed by both Catholic theologians and laymen mirror these changes in behavior [3; 4; 6]. In a national sample interviewed before and after Pope Paul's visit (October 1966) to the United Nations, 58% of the Catholics, compared with 55% of the non-Catholics, felt, before the Pope's visit, that the Catholic Church should ease its disapproval of contraceptive methods; directly after the Pope's visit, 55% of the Catholics and 52% of the non-Catholics still felt the same way. Catholic opinion was, however, influenced somewhat more than non-Catholic opinion by Pope Paul's statement at the United Nations calling upon the United Nations to ensure "enough bread on the tables of mankind and not to encourage artificial birth control."

There is, furthermore, no predictable relation between Catholic affiliation per se and birth rates. Some predominantly Catholic countries around the world exhibit very low birth rates.

[Note this sample of low birth rates among some countries that are more than 80% Catholic: Argentina (21.8), Belgium (16.4), France (17.7), Ireland (22.2), Luxembourg (15.6), Austria (17.9), and Italy (19.2). By comparison, the United States has a birth rate of 19.4 and Bulgaria, with the lowest among countries for which data is available, has 15.4. Ireland represents a special case in that this birth rate is achieved by delayed marriage and a low proportion of people married, methods that permit obedience to the Catholic doctrine concerning the use of contraceptives without, at the same time, experiencing rapid population growth. (Ireland's population is stable at present, partly because of out-migration.) Traditionally Catholic Latin American countries, with some exceptions, have very high birth rates with rates as high as 47–51 in the Dominican Republic, Ecuador, and Venezuela. (All of the birth rates cited in this essay represent number of births per thousand population; they are taken from the world population data sheet for 1966 compiled by the Population Reference Bureau in Washington, D.C.) In order to grasp the impact of such birth rates upon growth rates, one should note that these countries will double their populations in 20, 23, and 21 years respectively. These figures contrast sharply with countries like Belgium and Italy that will double their population in 117 and 100 years respectively.]

In view of these low birth rates in certain Catholic countries, we cannot explain the generally higher birth rates of Catholics as compared with Protestants within the same society simply by citing the Church's condemnation of contraceptives. (Ireland is an exception; Protestant Northern Ireland had a slightly higher birth rate in 1965 than Catholic Eire.)

Neither Hinduism nor Buddhism has any explicit teachings concerning the moral acceptability of contraceptives; Islam does, as we noted, officially approve their use. Nevertheless, this more official lack of opposition is not necessarily in accord with the religious beliefs held locally by great masses of people or even by some religious leaders. Reviewing what is known about the factors affecting fertility among the rural Sinhalese of Ceylon, Nag [35] notes that these Buddhists considered immoral the prevention of conception by means other than abstinence. Although some women expressed preferences for small families, almost all of them objected to any conscious attempt to prevent conception or birth. Nag describes the typical response as follows: "It is a great sin to try to prevent pregnancy. You must allow those to be born who are to be born" [35:47]. Men uniformly favored large families and wanted no control of births. Similar accounts have been given of the folk beliefs of followers of Islam. Edith Gates, recently retired from her position with the Pathfinder Fund, found that many Egyptian women did not know of the existing *fatwa* and believed that their religion forbade the use of contraceptives. Once advised of the *fatwa*, they were receptive to contraceptives and contraceptive advice.

Ryan [45] documented discrepancies among Ceylonese Buddhist Bhikku (priests) with respect to their moral assessment of contraception: the more educated tended to reconcile Buddhist principles with contraceptive practices; the less educated tended to find them irreconcilable. This same difference has been observed among Islamic religious leaders.

What about birth rates associated with these religions? Though Moslems have official permission to practice contraception, their birth rates are uniformly among the highest in the world. Two notable examples are Egypt (41–44) and Pakistan (49–53); Egypt is expected to double its population within 26 years, Pakistan in 22 years. No country in Asia has higher birth rates than Pakistan; a few countries in Africa exceed it but not by much. Among other major religious groups, Hindus are most comparable to the Moslems, but the Moslems of the Indian subcontinent have higher reproduction rates than their Hindu neighbors. India, 85% Hindu, has a birth rate of 40–43 and is expected to double its population in 31 years. Buddhist birth rates, according to Dudley Kirk [26], are more variable than those of Hindus and Moslems. In some countries, however, they are as high as the highest achieved by Moslems; note Burma (43–40) and Cambodia (47–53), countries due to double their population in 35 and 24 years respectively. Clearly the failure of these religions officially to condemn contraception is not correlated with low birth rates. As we pointed out earlier, even where, irrespective of folk beliefs, use of contraceptives has gained wide acceptance among Hindu and Moslem villagers of India and Pakistan, this factor by itself did not reduce the existing high birth rate.

It should be evident by now that, if we limit the study of the influence of religion upon fertility control to the influence exerted through promulgated doctrines and if among these doctrines we focus only upon those specifying acceptance or rejection of contraceptives, religion will not be interpreted as extremely important in understanding or solving the population problem. But religion has a much more significant and diverse relation to both fertility control and fertility rates.

Harvey Leibenstein has singled out the point at which fertility attitudes and practices must be changed if birth rates are to be sharply reduced. With startling directness, he reminds us of what should be obvious: "For the most part people have large families because they want them" [29:31]. *Desired* family size does not on the average deviate very much from *actual* family size. Whereas, in general, desired family size is higher than actual family size in developed countries, desired family size is lower than actual family size in underdeveloped countries. The difference between desired and actual family size in many of these underdeveloped countries is such that the introduction of perfect contraceptive knowledge and a perfect contraceptive device would reduce birth rates by less than 20%. The desired family size of the underdeveloped countries implies a doubling of the population roughly every generation and a very rapid population growth rate of more than 2% per year. The difference between desired and actual family size is considerably smaller than the difference between desired family size and replacement size. In order to reach a level at which the birth rate approximates the steady state death rate, birth rates in most underdeveloped countries like India and Pakistan would have to be reduced by more than 50%. Thus contraceptive control, without changes in motivation in the direction of desiring smaller families, cannot in underdeveloped countries result in birth rates that approach the steady state death rates. The felt-need hypothesis must definitely be supplemented by hypotheses concerning how we can increase the motivation to practice fertility control. What motivates us to want families of a certain size needs to be understood.

RELIGIOUS FACTORS AND OTHER FACTORS

Hypothetical analyses of factors related to increased fertility control have generally identified four sorts of situational inducements: considerable reductions in infant and child mortality; increased urbanization, industrialization, and the economic factors associated with these processes; a sense of group responsibility; and various kinds of education and information. In order to clarify more precisely the way in which religion relates to these inducements, it is essential to know what is entailed by the concept of *fertility control.*

So far this discussion of fertility control has been limited to the issues raised by the contraceptive techniques used to achieve some kind of control of birth rate. But "fertility control" refers more inclusively to public policy decisions about "population control" and to family planning by spacing births and controlling family size.

Many characterizations of religious positions have been confusing because they have lacked sophistication at this very juncture. Roman Catholics have generally, at the official level, opposed public population control although there are presently signs of change on this matter [52; 31]. Among the more thoughtful attempts at reformulation is that of Louis Dupré [15] as well as the three volumes resulting from the Notre Dame Conference on Population Problems edited by D.M. Barrett [3; 4]. Witness also Pope Paul VI's encyclical *Populorum Progressio* quoted in Dupré [15].

Family planning, however, has been condoned, even encouraged in the forms both of controlling size and spacing. The economic situation of the family and the health of the mother have been put forth as circumstances relevant to such planning. Catholic thought has stressed that family size must be determined by the family in its own circumstances and not by social or political agencies, not even by the Church.

[Family planning *in principle* was explicitly acknowledged in the frequently quoted passage from Pope Pius XII's Address to the Midwives, October 29, 1951: "Serious reasons often put forward on medical, eugenic, economic, and social grounds can exempt from that obligating service (the duty of providing for the conservation of the race) even for a considerable period of time, even for the entire duration of the marriage." However, the church has never delegated the authority, nor presumed to have the authority within itself to determine *when* such conditions exist. William Gibbons has observed that: "Unlike some advocates of planned parenthood, the Catholic Church has learned that ultimate decisions in this matter should be arrived at by the married people themselves" [20: 122]. Testifying before the House Committee on Foreign Affairs, Louis Dupré made this same point. While acknowledging that information and technical means for family planning should be made available to all, he nevertheless insisted that "the right to determine the size of the family belongs to the family alone" [15:7].]

It is fair to add, however, that the Church does promote the moral desirability of large families where having a large family is within the means of the couple involved.

[This point is unfortunately completely lost by Westoff, Potter, and Sagi. In their attempt to pinpoint whether religion can be regarded as a predictor of fertility, the following question was posed: "As far as you know, does your religion take any stand on size of family? What?" When 72% of the "active" Catholics and 61% of the "other" Catholics said that their church took "no stand," the researchers leapt to the conclusion that their data could be regarded as "largely refuting the theory that rejection of birth control is perceived by the Catholic population to reflect an official encouragement of large families" [47:85].

As we have noted above, the Catholic Church has been very careful to *avoid* specifying what family size ought to be. One "proper" answer to the ambiguous question posed in the authors' survey should have been precisely the one made by 72% of the "active" Catholics. From this, however, one cannot infer, as the authors do, that this same 72% believes that the Roman Catholic Church does *not* encourage large families. In fact, quite the opposite is the case, as Judith Blake has clearly documented. Amassing relevant passages from marriage manuals which denigrate the small family on the one hand and which eulogize the large family on the other as well as pertinent papal statements that unquestionably underscore the large family ideal, she concludes that: "So completely does this goal appear to pervade Catholic mass media, standard Catholic marriage manuals and the reward systems in Catholic culture that it hardly seems subject to misinterpretation" [7:27]. She observes also that, "during a ten year period ending in 1963, the mean family size of the Catholic Mother of the Year was 8.2 children. None of the mothers had fewer than five children and half had nine or ten offspring" [7:32].]

In the endeavor to specify the way in which religion affects the motivation to practice fertility control, a distinction has to be made between controlling birth intervals (spacing) and controlling family size. It is virtually meaningless to ask whether any given religion or culture does or does not favor or practice family planning. Spacing as a form of planning appears to be a more or less universal phenomenon. It has the sanction of religion because it helps to safeguard the health of mothers. A variety of traditional methods, especially breast feeding and restrictions upon intercourse, have served this purpose. The ready acceptance of modern contraceptives by people of various religions and cultures may very likely be bound up with the desire to increase the efficiency of spacing and thereby more predictably assist the mother to maintain her energy and health; one cannot, however, assume that those who accept contraceptives for these reasons will wish also deliberately to limit the size of their families beyond the limits set by the demands for spacing. In a personal communication, the Egyptian anthropologist Laila Shukry El Hamamsy has told of the Moslem peasant women who are shocked at even being asked whether they are trying to control the size of their families or to cease having children. Such matters are in God's hands. As the interviews and clinical experience show, these women have come to the birth clinic for a more dependable respite — offered by more efficient techniques — from the exhaustion of frequent childbearing.

Folk beliefs, religious and otherwise, do not uniformly condone or encourage self-conscious efforts to avoid having more than a certain number of children. Indeed, this is one of the most significant points at which religious variables become relevant for hypotheses that try to predict how motivation to control fertility can be increased. How, then, does religion affect the decisions to control family size? In somewhat "Tillichian" fashion, we prefer to think of religious beliefs as a fundamental value orientation to the whole of reality; religious beliefs entail a cognitive and emotional commitment to what is perceived to be of ultimate concern or value. Religious beliefs or belief systems can influence the person's perceptual and behavioral responses to his environment in at least two very basic ways: they induce the believer to have certain definite expectations of his environment both in the form of circumstances that permit the perpetuation of his religion through ritual and in the form of blessings or rewards for piety; secondly, they provide the believer with an orientation to the environment both in the form of more or less explicit views of the role of man and of God in shaping events in nature and in history and in the form of a stable pattern of responses, that is to say, in the form of a certain personality type. Each of these religiously prompted relations to one's environment has bearing in one way or another upon the motivation governing the decisions to control family size and, hence, upon actual birth rates.

One of the most critical rituals observed within Hinduism, demands that a father be buried by one of his sons. "The soul of a Hindu can depart in peace from its body only if the skull is opened by a son, who at the same time succeeds him as heir to the authority and obligations of his father" [32:153]. As long as relatively high mortality rates prevail, the religious requirement of a son who will survive and bury his father will serve as an incentive to have families large enough to provide "insurance" against the probable loss of some children. The realistic nature of such planning is forcefully brought home to us by the findings of Gordon and Wyon [50]: of the mothers they studied in the Punjab, half of those over 45 years old had lost a *minimum of three* live-born children. Under these circumstances, the reduction of mortality rates would seem to be a requisite condition for making reductions in family size feasible. Moslems also require sons for religious duties at and after death [26] and therefore experience the same kind of restraint upon limiting family size just ascribed to Hindus. Doctrinal injunctions to marry and multiply are found in all the major religions with the exception of Buddhism. Fagley [17] has given us a brief discussion of this in the major religions. The Protestant view on this is most thoroughly discussed in Fagley's *The Population Explosion and Christian Responsibility* [16]; the Catholic view, including ancient and medieval Christianity, in Noonan's *Contraception* [36].

For Moslems and Hindus, children and large families are among the highest blessings God can bestow. Buddhists also reflect the folk beliefs of the predominantly rural Moslem and

Hindu populations by putting a premium upon large families. In his study of Ceylonese priests, Ryan found that, "a minority of all priests believed that Buddhism directly supports the large family, although the view is rather widely held by the poorly educated. Thus slightly over half of the latter believed that the Buddha had favored large families of children over small, but only one of the (33) highly educated Bhikku agreed" [45:100]. The prevalence and significance of religious folk beliefs, including those of large numbers of relatively poorly educated religious leaders in the underdeveloped countries, needs to be better known and understood. Studies of this sort are increasing, however.

RELIGIOUS VALUES AND FAMILY SIZE

How potent and abiding are these religious values? What are the prospects for change in the direction of small family ideals? We have already seen that the reduction of mortality rates is, in any event, one of the motivational prerequisites for such changes. We must now consider the interaction between religious views of large families as blessings from God and the processes of urbanization and education, processes that demographers see as positive inducements to limit family size.

Demographers have generally maintained that, as urbanization increases, fertility rates decrease and, likewise, as education increases, fertility rates decrease. This overall pattern of association between urbanization or education on the one hand and fertility rates on the other has been observed in connection with the shift from high to low fertility rates, the demographic transition, in the West. This same pattern of association is now, to some degree, present in some of the less developed countries. Excellent reviews and analyses of the literature on this are to be found in Freedman [18] and more recently in Beshers [5].

With respect to the present differential in fertility between Catholics and Protestants in the United States, Beshers [5] expresses confidence that it will disappear once the Catholics have lived somewhat longer in the urban setting; similarly Judith

Blake [7] documents what she sees as a progressive "Americanization" of Catholic reproductive ideals. There is some evidence to suggest, however, that the Catholic to Protestant differential in fertility rates will, at least in the immediate future, persist, even increase, implying that the Catholic approbation of large families is retaining its influence.

[Whelpton, Campbell, and Patterson [48] apparently disagree with Beshers [5] and Blake [7]. As they interpret their data, the Protestant to Catholic differential in fertility is widening: Young Catholic wives expect more children than older Catholic wives; younger Protestant wives expect fewer than older Protestant wives. The authors specifically question the assumption that the differences between Catholics and non-Catholics will disappear once Catholics more nearly approximate the rest of the population in social and economic status because they found that the Catholic to Protestant differentials in family-size expectations are usually in the higher social and economic groups. This is, of course, what one would anticipate if Catholics are being obedient to the teachings of their Church; large families are only for those who can afford them. Time will tell whether *expected fertility* is, under prevailing conditions, a powerful enough predictor of actual fertility to prove the authors correct. Many fluctuating factors in the total environment can affect such a measure, and the effects upon Protestants and Catholics need not be the same. Changes in Catholic doctrine, for example, could be among them.

Westoff, Potter, and Sagi [47] found that the best predictor of higher Catholic rates was the amount of education in Catholic institutions, an indirect measurement of loyalty and involvement in the Church and of exposure to Catholic doctrine as well.]

But gross generalizations about the effects of urbanization and education upon fertility rates are not really extremely helpful. Where the so-called "western fertility pattern" is found in underdeveloped countries — where, in such countries, the better educated urban couples have considerably fewer children than their less educated rural counterparts — the educated urban group is so small that the overall birth rates are not greatly altered. India does not consistently exhibit the western fertility pattern; the Mysore study revealed the existence of this pattern but studies of Central India did not [5]. What is still more important is that speaking in this very general way of a "western fertility pattern" obscures some important facts about demographic behavior in both the East and the West. Paul Demeny [14] has found that low fertility within marriage first emerged on a large scale in Hungary within a *fundamentally peasant setting;* this occurred at a time when fertility within marriage was very high in the *cities* of the Austrian-Hungarian region. Regarding India, Kingsley Davis, in response to questions during a faculty seminar at Harvard in 1966, expressed profound doubt that urbanization and industrialization are having the expected effect on demographic behavior. According to Davis, England had attained a shift to markedly lower birth rates by the time it was as industrialized and as urban as India is now; India, however, shows no sign of such a shift in birth rates.

What is it about urbanization or education that has come to be generally associated with low fertility within marriage, but could be true of some peasant cultures and could also fail sometimes to be true in an urban setting, even sometimes among the educated? The following general conditions would meet these criteria: (1) circumstances in which there are decided advantages, both to the parents and to the children, in having few children in one family; (2) a mode of orientation toward one's circumstances that permits and facilitates rational and purposive responses to them. These conditions may not be sufficient to ensure small family size but they are among the *sine qua non* for making it desirable.

In an urbanizing and industrializing society, large families tend to be economic liabilities rather than assets; the labor of children is much less needed and their opportunities to become financially independent and successful tend to increase with the careful budgeting of their parents. In a money economy, in contrast to a subsistence economy, children are economic liabilities. Money is required for food, clothing, and education. Housing and living space are at a premium, and crowding is undesirable to parents and children alike. Careful budgeting can provide many special cultural and educational benefits, privileges, and opportunities for an urban family; children are a critical part of such budgeting. Small families tend to be mutually advantageous to parents and children under these conditions so typical of urban settings in the West.

But comparable conditions have arisen and do exist in rural settings as well, even in peasant cultures. In rural areas, land of a financially viable size can become extremely scarce. Coupled with the absence of alternative economic and vocational opportunities, a situation is created that one could very well describe as "population pressure." Of two different castes living in the same villages of the Punjab region of India, the farming caste had a relatively lower fertility rate than the leather-worker caste [39]. This same farming caste limited also the number of married sons in order to avoid an undue fragmentation of their farms. Fertility rates, however, even for the farming caste were still high; wives aged 45 and over averaged 7.0 live births. Yet the members of this caste seemed already to be making rational and purposive responses to their particular situation. On the basis of intensive research in this region of India, Gordon and Wyon [50] have hypothesized that people in such an area would be motivated to reduce their birth rates if: mortality rates for infants and children were sharply decreased; local social units were stimulated to measure their own population dynamics and to draw inferences from them concerning their own welfare and aspirations; and efficient methods of birth control were introduced. Introducing these conditions would substantially increase the opportunities of each family unit to reduce family size without undue fear, to assess in a more exact and realistic way how fertility goals would affect themselves and their community, and to plan with more realistic hopes for success in attaining their goals. Whether birth rates would be markedly lowered by bringing about these conditions alone would depend not simply upon the extent to which people in that region start to benefit from such a reduction but also upon the extent to which people actually perceive such benefits and believe that they are attainable.

The gathering of vital statistics is, therefore, crucial: Not until statistics were introduced did the first vaccines gain general acceptance in the West. Without accurate information, a sense of group responsibility cannot exist on a rational basis and will have no perceptible dividend to the individual members. The eventual achievement of "replacement level" fertility rates through the voluntary exercise of fertility control is contingent upon providing the conditions for perceiving the desirability of that level.

The proposal of Gordon and Wyon for the Punjab assumes that rational and purposive behavior more or less exists already and can be intensified by modifications in the environment which make the intensification of such behavior more beneficial and more attainable. This assumption is plausible enough and may very well turn out to be justified, at least for certain regions and cultures.

But modes of orientation to life, and the personality types associated with them, have a hardy and independent existence of their own. And, as we noted previously, they have their say in determining how the circumstances of our lives will look to us and what kinds of responses we consider appropriate to various events in nature and in history.

It is one thing to try to make people aware, when the situation warrants it, of the benefits of planning a small family. It is quite another to try to elicit the control of family size per se where *exerting such control* is viewed as grossly impious, unmanly, or undesirable.

Our orientation to nature and to historical circumstances is very much bound up with our understanding of the relationship of man's actions to the powers that shape events in nature and in history. Florence Kluckhohn [27] has specified the following five basic value orientations that order and direct the solutions to problems that must be solved by peoples at all times and places: (1) the orientation to human nature; (2) the orientation to the relation of man to nature (and supernature) — the man-nature orientation; (3) the orientation to time; (4) the orientation to human activity; and (5) the orientation to man's relationship to other men. At present we are discussing (2) and shortly we shall take up (3).

Beliefs concerning God's active sphere of dominion and participation in human affairs directly affect attitudes toward controlling family size and define the limits of propriety with respect to taking matters into one's own hands. Thus, as Richard Fagley has noted,

> A principal pro-natalist factor in Islam stems from a strong belief in the active providence of Allah. It is Allah who creates sexuality and determines procreation or barrenness. . . . A tradition quotes the Prophet as saying, "whichever soul is destined to come to this world shall come." This concept of predestination gives a strong sense of *kismet*, fate, to the ethos of Islam, which undoubtedly does much to sustain high fertility patterns. Since it includes trust in the beneficent character of divine providence, any question of restricting the number of offspring tends to appear as lacking in piety [17:81].

These beliefs in the will of Allah do indeed find their expression in folk piety. Rural Moslems speak of having as many children as God wills and restrict the use of contraceptives, where they are used, to the demands of spacing. Hinduism and Buddhism have doctrines of *ahimsa*, noninjury, and of the cycle of *karma*, the law of cause and effect or of sowing and reaping in human affairs. In the popular mind, the conscious endeavor to prevent a conception or a birth other than by abstinence has often been interpreted as injury to life and as an interference in natural and morally inviolable cosmic processes.

Interesting parallels to these religious beliefs can be found in certain subcultures. The Gaucho of South America, who works on ranches as a cowboy, considers it unmanly to take rational forethought. For him, rational forethought is cowardly, a failure to face what "life" or "fate" has in store for each of us. Some coeds in the United States play a kind of Russian roulette by deliberately refusing to use contraceptives, claiming that thereby they obtain an "authentic sexual experience." Among working-class wives in the United States there is a tendency described by Lee Rainwater [40] to be sceptical of thinking and planning ahead.

Each of these orientations to the environment shares one very important ingredient: the tendency to eschew, for one reason or another, the future-time perspective characteristic of the purposive-rational type of personality. This personality type was first identified by Max Weber. In *The Protestant Ethic and the Spirit of Capitalism* Weber traced the religious origins of this type of personality within Calvinism and espoused the thesis that the origin of such a personality type was an essential part of the development of the social system that precipitated and sustained capitalism. Banks [1] has noted the critical role of this future-time oriented, budgeting, type of person for bringing down fertility rates within marriage in Victorian England. Lately both Banks [2] and Beshers [5] have called attention to the significance of this personality type for favoring and actualizing small family ideals. They also make the point that future-time orientation is an ingredient of religious belief within Christianity; Banks [2] develops a plausible set of hypotheses regarding the mechanisms by which Christianity gives rise to the rationalistic-purposive orientation.

Beshers [5] maintains that there are three types of social constraints upon decision-making about family size within the family unit: mode of orientation to time (personality type); budget calculation; and communication within the family. The first and second factors are combined in the purposive-rational personality type. Beshers finds also that there are three basic personality types differentiated by their future-time orientation: traditional; short-run hedonistic; and purposive-rational. The traditional personality type tends to be oriented to the past and is not prone to make use of new information for assessing the present or looking to the future. Rural Moslems, Buddhists, and, perhaps to a somewhat lesser extent, Hindus tend to exhibit this mode of orientation. The Gauchos, the coeds, and the working class in the United States tend toward the short-run hedonistic type of orientation. Both types, as we noted above, are deficient in the future-time perspective of the purposive-rational type, lacking therefore the predisposition to plan and budget for the future and to limit family size in accord with such calculations.

The religious origins, within Christianity, of the purposive-rational mode of orientation, have already been mentioned.

Especially significant for the development of this type of person were Calvin's doctrines of providence and of vocation. Every act of man had a purpose in God's scheme and, what is still more important, every action of man was a joint venture in achieving God's purpose for man and the whole cosmos. Through purposive and rational activity man could share in the mighty works of God in nature and in history. By such activities, a man could gain assurance of divine favor and of participation in a community of faith and purpose within which membership was not determined by blood relationships or geographical origins. This community was seen to have a glorious future — one of brotherhood and equity — which could be secured only by diligent and efficient dominion over the goods of this earth.

Weber believed that the purposive-rational personality type needed this ideological basis for its origin but that, once bureaucratic structures arose, they would in turn perpetuate the personality type. Hence the process often called "secularization" is set in motion and a purposive-rational pattern of behavior persists without explicit religious rationalization.

Critical questions, therefore, arise about the possibilities of fostering universally the kind of behavior characteristic of the purposive-rational personality spawned in western society. If such behavior is to be induced, will it be necessary, both morally and practically, for the people of nonwestern countries to find the resources for fostering it within their own great religious traditions? Or will economic development by itself create bureaucratic structures that will by themselves elicit the desired personality type? Since the religious and value systems of these countries are not directly comparable to those within which bureaucratization took place in the West, the answers to these questions are not clear.

It is possible that, at least in some societies, the conditions posited above in the Gordon-Wyon hypothesis will suffice. Certainly they represent certain *sine qua non* for making the control of family size a rationally feasible enterprise. In any event, demographers and others concerned with the population problem must learn much more about religious beliefs at the folk level and must learn to respect both their motivating power and their appropriateness to the settings within which they occur. In every religious tradition God is conceived as being on the side of his people, and, when many children are needed, God favors his people. Calvinism, with its emphasis on man as a coworker with God, could easily shift from the blessings of the large family to the blessing of relatively few well-educated, prosperous children with a future. One should not presume that other major religions cannot make similar adjustments.

We have now completed an assessment of the felt-need hypothesis and of hypotheses as to how the motivation to control fertility within marriage can be increased. Now we wish only briefly to touch upon the third contemporary type of variation on Malthus' hypothesis that Moral Restraint (plus or minus Misery and Vice) determines the birth rate, limiting ourselves to those measures concerned with the postponement of the age of marriage of women.

When the average age of marriage of women is increased, birth rates are reduced. This is true because the average length of the fertile period is shortened while the age-specific fertility rate after marriage does not appreciably rise. Delayed marriage, along with low proportions of married women, were initially important for the demographic transition in the West.

Postponement of marriage, apart from its general significance for western birth rates, including in a very special way those of Ireland, can be expected to help lower fertility rates in a number of underdeveloped countries. Wyon et alia [49] have documented this for India. There is a trend toward later marriages in what Dudley Kirk [26] calls "the more progressive Moslem countries." In such countries, postponement of marriage can be accelerated by providing women greater independence and self-confidence, and improved status outside of marriage. Accomplishing this requires better education of girls and enlarged opportunities for employment for girls and women outside the home. The provision of education for women would tend also to induce the purposive-rational pattern of behavior needed for efficiently controlling fertility.

MARXIST AND CATHOLIC POLICIES

We have yet to examine the Marxist and Catholic response to Malthus. In both of these instances, the whole idea of "overpopulation" was rejected. Marxists and Catholics alike initially objected to any explicit attempt on the part of governments to control or seek to control population growth. The classic Marxian formulation of the problem of population is found in Engels' "Outlines of a Critique of Political Economy" (1844):

> The area of land is limited, — that is perfectly true. But the labour power to be employed on this area increases together with the population; and even if we assume that the increase of labour is not always proportionate to the latter, there still remains a third element — which the economists, however, never consider as important — namely, science, the progress of which is just as limitless and at least as rapid as that of population . . . in the most normal conditions it also grows in geometrical progression — and what is impossible for science?

Although the Chinese communists have adhered rigidly to this Marxian assertion that "overpopulation" per se can never exist in the socialist state and that any inequity in resources as over against demand — what Catholics often refer to as "relative overpopulation" — is but a consequence of the capitalist mode of production, nevertheless the Chinese have demonstrated a marked capacity for flexibility with regard to the question of birth control. Thus, whereas official policy concerning birth control has undergone more than one volte-face in the last decade, Malthus' theory is consistently rejected. Arguments justifying the restriction of family size are invoked such as "the protection of women and children . . . the up-bringing and education of the rising generation . . . and the health and prosperity of the nation" (speech by Chou-en-lai, September 1956) as well as insisting on sexual equality and the need to devote one's energies to the development of the state. These restrictions include such measures as mandatory late marriages (men must be 30, women 25) and severe sanctions against having more than two children per couple.

Like the Chinese, the Russians have retained the traditional, categorical rejection of malthusian and neomalthusian thought while at the same time implying by their policies that the regulation of the size and growth of population is well within the scope of governmental authority [22].

The classical Catholic óbjections to Malthus as well as the shift to more realistic responses can, appropriately enough, be documented by reference to separate statements by Pope Paul VI. In the first statement made at the United Nations on October 1965, the Pope called for food for the hungry rather than programs to encourage contraception.

[Zimmerman quotes a strong expression of the conservative Catholic reaction to public encouragement of family planning: "The Church has never advised an individual *family* and much less a whole nation to use the Rhythm method . . . . The organizations that recommend birth limitation on a large scale, it does not matter under what form, are relying upon the erroneous opinion that the family is for the State. It is the contrary that is true: the State is for the family and it cannot be admitted that the family must, in its most intimate life, submit itself to considerations of a demographic nature. The State, on the contrary, must assure all families of the country of the possibility of providing a becoming livelihood and education not only for one or two children but for the normal family as willed by God. To save a nation from the threat of famine it is possible to see solutions other than of limiting births, no matter how this is accomplished" [52:204–205].]

In the Pope's later statement, contained in the encyclical *Populorum Progressio*, the problems associated with rapid population growth, as well as the urgency of government policies with respect to it, are acknowledged and a plea is made for preserving the voluntary nature of family planning.

[It is true that too frequently an accelerated demographic increase adds its own difficulties to the problems of development: the size of the population increase more rapidly than available resources, and things are found to have reached apparently an impasse. From that moment the temptation is great to check the demographic increase by means of radical measures. It is certain that public authorities can intervene, within the limit of their competence by favoring the availability of appropriate information and by adopting suitable measures, provided that these be in conformity with the moral law and that they respect the rightful freedom of married couples. Where the inalienable right to marriage and procreation is lacking, human dignity has ceased to exist. Finally, it is for the parents to decide with full knowledge of the matter, on the number of their children.]

No more than Marxism has Catholicism prevented governmental contributions to family planning. In 1966 the Agency for International Development contributed $5.5 million toward the support of family planning programs in Pakistan, Turkey, South Korea, Jamaica, and, significantly, in the primarily Roman Catholic Latin American nations of Brazil, Costa Rica, Ecuador, El Salvador, and Honduras. Futhermore, lay Catholic opinion is keeping pace with the shift in official thought. A Gallup Poll taken in October 1965 revealed that a majority of the Roman Catholics in the United States supports the idea of Federal aid for family planning clinics.

The Catholic insistence upon the voluntary nature of decisions regarding family size is a most laudatory one. Although it is not always easy to discover why, in a given region, a sense of group responsibility for population growth is essential, efforts must be made to discern and make known any erosion of the quality of our lives due to population pressures. And, as we have argued earlier, if we are to evoke voluntary reductions of family size which are in accord with the needs of one's population group, we must not only learn to work with and respect the particular circumstances of that region, but also learn to respect the potentiality of the cultural and religious heritage of these groups for working out the most viable and likely sources of deep and abiding motivation to accomplish such reductions of family size and, hence, of rapid population growth.

REFERENCES

1. Banks, J A: *Prosperity and Parenthood* (Routledge & Kegan Paul, Ltd, London, England) 1954.
2. Banks, J A: Historical Sociology and the Study of Population, *Daedalus* (paper presented at the International Conference on Historical Population Studies, Bellagio, Italy) forthcoming.
3. Barrett, Donald N, ed: *The Problem of Population*, vol 1, 2 (University of Notre Dame Press, Notre Dame, Indiana) 1964.
4. Barrett, Donald N: *The Problem of Population*, vol 3 (University of Notre Dame Press, Notre Dame, Indiana) 1965.
5. Beshers, James M: *Population Processes in Social Systems* (The Free Press, New York, New York) 1967.
6. Birmingham, William, ed: *What Modern Catholics Think about Birth Control* (Signet Books, The New American Library, Inc, New York, New York) 1964.
7. Blake, Judith: The Americanization of Catholic Reproductive Ideals, *Population Studies*, vol 20, 1966, pp 27–43.
8. Bogue, Donald J: The Demographic Breakthrough: from Projection to Control, *Population Index*, vol 30, 1964, pp 449–454.
9. Cobb, John C; Raulet, Harry M; and Harper, Paul: An I.U.D. Field Trial in Lulliani, West Pakistan (paper presented at the American Public Health Association) Oct 21, 1965.
10. Coale, Ansley J: The Decline of Fertility in Europe from the French Revolution to World War II, *Daedalus* (paper presented at the International Conference on Historical Population Studies, Bellagio, Italy) forthcoming.
11. Cox, Harvey: *The Secular City* (The Macmillan Company, New York, New York) 1965.
12. Davis, Kingsley: Values, Population, and the Supernatural: A Critique, in G F Mair, ed: *Studies in Population* (Prince-

ton University Press, Princeton, New Jersey) 1949, p 137.

13. Davis, Kingsley: Fertility Control and the Demographic Transition in India, *The Interrelations of Demographic, Economic, and Social Problems in Selected Underdeveloped Areas* (Milbank Memorial Fund, New York, New York) 1954.

14. Demeny, Paul: Some Factors Associated with the Early Decline of Marital Fertility in Austria-Hungary, *Daedalus* (paper presented at the International Conference on Historical Population Studies, Bellagio, Italy) forthcoming.

15. Dupré, Louis: in Chakerian, Charles G, and Dupré, Louis: *Two Theological Views on Population Control* (Population Reference Bureau, Inc, selection no 21) reprinted from *McCormick Quarterly*, vol 20, no 2, Jan 1967.

16. Fagley, Richard M: *The Population Explosion and Christian Responsibility* (Oxford University Press, New York, New York) 1960.

17. Fagley, Richard M: Doctrines and Attitudes of Major Religions in Regard to Fertility, *World Population Conference, 1965*, vol 2 (United Nations, New York, New York) 1967.

18. Freedman, Ronald: The Sociology of Human Fertility, *Current Sociology* (Basil Blackwell) vol 10/11, 1963, pp 35 – 121.

19. Freedman, Ronald; Whelpton, Pascal K; and Campbell, Arthur A: *Family Planning, Sterility, and Population Growth* (McGraw-Hill Book Company, New York, New York) 1959.

20. Gibbons, William J: The Catholic Value System in Relation to Human Fertility in G F Mair, ed: *Studies in Population* (Princeton University Press, Princeton, New Jersey) 1949, p 138.

21. Hauser, Philip M, ed: *The Population Dilemma* (Prentice-Hall, Inc, Englewood Cliffs, New Jersey) 1963.

22. Heer, David: Abortion, Contraception, and Population Policy in the Soviet Union, *Soviet Studies*, vol 17, 1965, pp 76–83.

23. Henry, Louis: Some Data on Natural Fertility, *Eugenics Quarterly*, vol 8, 1961, pp 81–91.

24. Himes, Norman E: *Medical History of Contraception* (Gamut Press, Taplinger Publishing Co, Inc, New York, New York) 1963.

25. Kirk, Dudley: Prospects for Reducing Natality in the Underdeveloped World, *The Annals of the American Academy of Political and Social Science*, vol 369, Jan 1967, pp 48–60.

26. Kirk, Dudley: Factors Affecting Moslem Natality, *World Population Conference, 1965*, vol 2 (United Nations, New York, New York) 1967.

27. Kluckhohn, Florence, and Strodtbeck, Fred L: *Variations in Value Orientations* (Row, Peterson & Co, now Harper & Row, Publishers, New York, New York) 1961.

28. Langer, Elinor: in *Science*, Dec 10, 1965, p 1433, quoting an editorial in the *Washington Post*.

29. Leibenstein, Harvey: Population Growth and the Development of Underdeveloped Countries, *Harvard Medical Alumni Bulletin*, vol 41, 1967, pp 29–33.

30. Lenski, Gerhard: *The Religious Factor* (Doubleday and Company, Inc, Garden City, New York) 1961.

31. Lestapis, Stanislas de: *Family Planning and Modern Problems* (Herder and Herder, New York, New York) 1961.

32. Lorimer, Frank: *Culture and Human Fertility* (I.F.M.R.P., Unesco, Paris, France) 1954.

33. Malthus, Thomas Robert: *On Population, 1798 and 1803* (Modern Library, Inc, New York, New York), 1960.

34. Mudd, Stuart, ed: *The Population Crisis and the Use of World Resources* (Indiana University Press, Bloomington, Indiana) 1964.

35. Nag, Moni: *Factors Affecting Human Fertility in Nonindustrial Societies: A Cross-Cultural Study* (Yale University Press, New Haven, Connecticut) 1962.

36. Noonan, John T, jr: *Contraception* (The Belknap Press of Harvard University Press, Cambridge, Massachusetts) 1965.

37. Novak, Michael: *The Experience of Marriage* (The Macmillan Company, New York, New York) 1964.

38. Potter, Ralph B: Religion, Politics, and Population: A Time

for Change, *Harvard Medical Alumni Bulletin*, vol 41, 1967, pp 14–21.

39. Potter, Robert G, jr; New, Mary L; Wyon, John B; and Gordon, John E: A Fertility Differential in Eleven Punjab Villages, *Milbank Memorial Fund Quarterly*, vol 43, Apr 1965, pp 185–201.

40. Rainwater, Lee; Coleman, Richard P; and Handel, Gerald: *Workingman's Wife* (Oceana Publications, Inc, Dobbs Ferry, New York) 1959.

41. Revelle, Roger: The Problem of People, *Harvard Today*, Autumn 1965, pp 2–9.

42. Revelle, Roger: Population and Food Supplies: the Edge of the Knife, *Proceedings of the National Academy of Sciences*, vol 56, 1966, pp 328–351.

43. Rizk, Hanna: Social and Psychological Factors Affecting Fertility in the United Arab Republic, *Marriage and Family Living*, vol 25, no 1, Feb 1963.

44. Ross, John A: Recent Events in Population Control, *Studies in Family Planning* (a publication of The Population Council) no 9, 1966, pp 1–5.

45. Ryan, Bryce: Hinayana Buddhism and Family Planning in Ceylon, in *The Interrelations of Demographic, Economic, and Social Problems in Selected Underdeveloped Areas* (Milbank Memorial Fund, New York, New York) 1954.

46. Thompson, Warren S, and Lewis, David T: *Population Problems* (McGraw-Hill Book Company, Inc, New York, New York) 1965.

47. Westoff, Charles F; Potter, Robert G, jr; and Sagi, Philip C: *The Third Child* (Princeton University Press, Princeton, New Jersey) 1963.

48. Whelpton, Pascal K; Campbell, Arthur A; and Patterson, John E: *Fertility and Family Planning in the United States* (Princeton University Press, Princeton, New Jersey) 1966.

49. Wyon, John B; Finner, Stephen L; Heer, David M; Parthasarathy, Nadipurum R; and Gordon, John E: Delayed Marriage and Prospects for Fewer Births in Punjab Villages, *Demography*, vol 3, no 1, 1966, pp 209–217.

50. Wyon, John B, and Gordon, John E: The Khanna Study, *Harvard Medical Alumni Bulletin*, vol 41, 1967, pp 24–28.
51. Wyon, J B, and Gordon, J E: *The Khanna Population Study* (Harvard University Press, Cambridge, Massachusetts) forthcoming.
52. Zimmerman, Anthony: *Catholic Viewpoint on Overpopulation* (Hanover House, Garden City, New York) 1961.

7. WHAT IS THE VALUE OF LIFE?

by Herbert W. Richardson

WHAT IS THE VALUE of life? Reverse the question: When is life utterly without value? When is life worthless?

A man lies in a hospital bed. His heartbeat is maintained by artificial stimulation and his brain has by now lost all reactive power. His illness is irreversible. He will never again regain consciousness. Why do we hesitate to pull the switch?

A fetus is growing beneath the heart of a woman who dreams of imminent motherhood. But her dreams will become nightmares. The baby growing inside her is defective. It will never learn to say "Mama"; it will never learn to tie its shoes; it will never know it is a human person. What value can such life have? Why not abort it before we look upon its face?

The lives of the patient in the hospital and the defective fetus seem to be valueless because they lack all capacity to enjoy even minimum human fulfillment. They will never experience the happiness of joys remembered, of love shared, of things hoped for and attained. *The first value of life, then, is in all those things that contribute to human happiness.*

But there is something more in life than happiness and its pursuit.

Imagine that you are a doctor engaged in cancer research. You care for a ward of patients, now elderly and senile, who are in the last stages of various terminal illnesses. Their lives are as good as over. They shall experience no further human fulfillment and shall bring no more joy into the lives of their friends or family. But you could use them in such a way that mankind might benefit. You could inject cells into their bodies in order to study the effects. Such an experiment would probably not shorten their lives and might lead to immense good.

Several years ago such an experiment was performed on terminal patients in a New York hospital. The doctors involved were not discharged for appreciably shortening the lives of their patients. They were discharged because they violated a basic human value, a value which conflicted with the desire to increase the happiness of all mankind. They were discharged for performing this experiment upon their patients without the patients' consent — a basic ethical principle governing medical research.

The principle of informed consent was formulated at Nuremburg after the Second World War as a specification of the wrong done by German doctors who used concentration camp prisoners for medical experimentation. These doctors reasoned in a humanitarian way. They knew that the prisoners were marked for an early death and that they themselves were utterly helpless to prevent this or ameliorate their condition. In principle, the prisoners were as good as dead and, separated from all friends and family, now experienced only the torment of anticipating their doom. Since these prisoners were going to die anyway, the doctors reasoned, why not take advantage of the situation to benefit all mankind? Why not use them for medical experimentation?

Why not? Because there is another value to life besides the happiness of mankind and its increase; because the greatest happiness of the greatest number cannot justify to any individual the denial of the right to decide about the use of his body; because if all the happiness in the world could be bought for the price of selling even one person into involuntary servitude, that happiness would be immoral. To reject the right of a man to choose his own fate is to sacrifice a value that outweighs happiness itself.

We see, then, that the endurance of suffering may be right when the alleviation of that unhappiness can only be accomplished by violating human dignity, by sacrificing human freedom and truth. This was the heroic affirmation of the portrait of Thomas More in *A Man For All Seasons*. He shows us a second basic value of life, *the value of human freedom*.

But what about those who lack the capacity to decide for themselves? Isn't this precisely the situation of the terminally ill patient or the human fetus? Someone else must decide for them as well as for all minors who because of youth, illness, or other incapacity are unable to understand their situations and are without the ability to choose. Minors are fully human, but need our special care. Because of their minority, their weakness, we must choose in their behalf. Moreover, because of their weakness, it is always presumed that *the caring exercise of choice on behalf of a minor always will involve some special advantage to him and some special disadvantage to the one who is stronger and is responsible for acting on his behalf.*

Suppose, for example, you know a parent whose choices respecting his children always work out to his own advantage rather than to theirs. Is he really caring for them or is he taking advantage of their weakness and using them as things? Or suppose you are a wife who must decide whether your incurably ill husband should continue to be kept alive. If your decision is to your own advantage, then how can you be sure that you are really caring for *him?*

It is because of this disequilibrium of advantage characteristic of true caring that we especially revere, protect, even "uselessly prolong" the lives of the weak: the terminally ill patient, the mentally retarded, the little child. The mark of a caring person or society is the protection and special advantage it accords to the weak, to those unable to fend for themselves.

The life for which we care is the life whose destiny we regard as intertwined with our own. When we identify with others we suffer with them in their place. This feeling of identification with others is the foundation of all compassion (*compassio*, to suffer together) and moral action. It is alluded to in the Great Commandment and in the golden rule of every religion: "Do unto others as you would have them do unto you." That is, imagine yourself in their place, identify with them, feel how you participate together in a single life.

The "golden rule" feeling of identification is the presupposition of all ethical behavior. This is because we only treat with respect that life which we first acknowledge, or recognize, as bound up with our own. Because of this feeling of identification, we act towards others as if they were ourselves. This is why every moral obligation is both an obligation to another and an obligation to oneself. More exactly, every moral obligation is a single obligation towards · one whole reality to which I and others belong.

REVERENCE FOR LIFE

The feeling of unity, or sense of participation with others in a larger whole, is technically called reverence for life. Some people seem to have very little of this reverence for life or fellow feeling. They identify only with a small group of others — sometimes only with their family or racial group, sometimes only with a somewhat more abstract social unit such as their nation. And it may be that there are some people who identify with nothing outside of themselves, having absolutely no fellow feeling. In this case they will be called amoral. For they do not experience that motivational reality on which all particular ethical actions depend. Because reverence for life is the root of all particular ethical actions, it therefore must be enumerated among the values of life.

Hence we now enumerate three: (1) *the value of happiness* (including all the things we use to make us happy), (2) *the value of freedom* (including the intellectual understanding that makes choice possible), and (3) *the value of reverence for life* (including the care that expresses it).

Reverence for life is a matter of both extensiveness and intensiveness. It relates not only to the number of beings for whom we care, but also to the degree of care we feel for each of them. Most of us care more about those to whom we are related by ties of blood than to all others; next we care more about those we know in person than those we do not know personally. This is why we are more grieved by injuries that befall our family and acquaintances than by injuries that befall persons whom we know only through the newspapers. For even though we may feel some small compassion for those we have never met, we usually identify with them less and so care about them less.

For most of us, therefore, the feeling of reverence for life can be diagrammed as a circular area that is very intense at the center (ourselves, family, close friends) while becoming increasingly less intense toward the edges where it shades off almost indiscernibly into that area of life with which we feel absolutely no identification and for which we do not care at all. On the penumbral fringes of this circle, huddled just barely within it, are many of the weak: the mentally retarded, the physically disabled, the genetically defective, the seriously ill, primitive and aboriginal peoples, and even our enemies. They all seem to lack certain characteristics that we feel are essential to ourselves and so we identify with them only slightly — and sometimes not at all.

Today we should recall that many of those who huddle in this penumbra of humanity have, until recently, been regarded as nonsacred expendable life. In fact, it is only within the last two hundred years that members of other races, women, and even children have been regarded as more than property. And though we seem, at last, to have agreed about their status as fully human beings, we argue still about the status of the terminally ill and the human fetus. When a patient's brain is no longer reactive, then may we use the rest of his body as a mine from which to obtain transplant organs? And what of the fetus? Should we care for it as a weaker human life, accepting the fact that such choosing in its behalf always must involve a disequilibrium of advantage in its favor?

The difficulty of settling these questions arises from a conflict among the values of happiness, freedom, and reverence for life. Apart from this conflict between our happiness and our continued care for the life of a human fetus or someone terminally ill, we would find no special difficulty in allowing such weaker life to exist. For apart from this conflict, the continued existence of such life would in no way disadvantage us or limit our freedom. But when there is such a conflict, we are pressed to a choice among the competing values. Should we accept disadvantage and limit our freedom by the continued preservation of such life or should we limit our fellow feeling and sense of identification with such life in order to enhance our happiness and opportunities for choice?

A conflict of values can take place both within an individual self and within a larger society of persons. Such a conflict threatens to disintegrate them and hence must be resolved in order for there to be a personal or social unity and identity. The right resolution of a potential conflict among several values is called justice. Justice is both the harmonizing power of the several tendencies of the inner spirit of a man (a just man) and the ordering principle of an entire society (a just society).

Because justice aims at the maximization of values through their harmonization, it is a value in itself. Hence, to the list we have been enumerating we now add: (4) *the value of justice* (including all the ordering resources of life).

Notice that justice is not simply an ordering of external relations and behavior. It is also an ordering of various values, attitudes, and tendencies within the inner person. Such "psychological justice" is the principle that seeks to harmonize and actualize the full range of valuings that a person feels — his desire for maximal happiness, his desire for maximal freedom, and his desire for maximal unity with other beings.

Justice is rooted in the demand of the self (or of a society, if we think of social justice) for integration. A person's inner life is ordered and oriented in a definite way, whether he accomplishes this himself or passively accepts the person-forming influences from his society and culture. The conflict of values at stake in any particular problem (e.g., abortion) is not, therefore, simply a conflict that exists between persons, but is also a conflict of feelings that exists within a person.

Someone who claims that the fetus is simply a tumorous blob of tissue having no right to life is ordering his own inner feelings and his psychological life in a definite way. Such a claim could only be made by *a certain kind of person.* Whether abortion is right or not is therefore not simply a question about social justice, but a question about psychological justice. It is a question about the kinds of people we want to be. Are persons most just as persons, have they maximally actualized and harmonized the full range of values when they order their inner life by refusing to identify with and reverence fetal life? The same question can be raised with regard to persons who achieve psychological integration by refusing to identify with persons of other races, or nationalities, or even of the opposite sex. Are such persons as truly persons when they achieve their psychological integration by diminishing the range of values they affirm? Don't persons who achieve psychological integration in this way not only lack justice in their actions, but also in their very soul? Aren't they somewhat less as persons than a person ought to be?

Justice is rooted in the demand of any self or society for order and integration and it must fulfill this demand. But merely to order and to integrate is not, ipso facto, justice. There can be law and order that is unjust. Justice must not only order the values of life (including all the behavior that expresses value), but must order them in such a way that all value claims are maximally and simultaneously coaffirmed.

RELATIVE JUSTICE

Justice always aims at perfect harmony, that is, at a simultaneous affirmation of value claims in such a way that none must be sacrificed. This perfect justice is so difficult to achieve, however, that we usually must compromise for the best possible combination of compatible values. Such a compromise order is called "relative justice." *Because it always involves the rejection of some values for the sake of affirming others, a relatively just compromise is also relatively unjust. For the sake of justice, therefore, men and societies are frequently required to tolerate injustice.*

It may be relatively just to organize society in terms of a reverence for the sanctity of all life. But in India, where sacred cows are fed while children starve, it is also relatively unjust. It

may be relatively just for a benevolent dictatorship to deny freedom to its citizens while seeking to promote and increase their
happiness; but this denial of freedom is also an injustice. And it
may be relatively just, in American society, to organize life in
terms of a maximization of the value of freedom. But we should
also see how this identification of justice with freedom has provided the rhetoric used to justify a disregard for the lives of the
weak. In the name of freedom America has decimated the Indian, the Negro, the ghetto dweller, the Appalachian poor, and
most recently, the people of Vietnam. By focusing our ethical
rhetoric on the justification for the destruction of these peoples,
we have failed to see how the "justice of freedom" perpetrates
vast injustice and violence to the sanctity of life. For a relative
justice is also an injustice.

We should ask ourselves, in view of America's traditional disregard for the sanctity of life as a part of the value mix, whether
our present willingness to exclude the human fetus and the terminally ill patient from that community of life with which we
feel we are a part is not one more manifestation of our national
pathology. It is a pathological state of affairs when a person or
society has so identified its particular compromise of value claims
with perfect justice that it no longer sees the injustice which it
perpetrates in the name of justice.

Injustice can and usually does seek to justify itself by adduc-
ing as its legitimate reason for existing the correlative values affirmed in the compromise of a value conflict. It can always do
this. Since no values are ever repudiated and overruled except
for the sake of maintaining or increasing other values, injustice
is always found in conjunction with relative justice and is always
perpetrated out of a desire to attain some good. This leads to *a
consistent rhetoric of injustice* wherein persons constantly call
attention to the positive values in any given compromise and
suggest that the evil which this compromise accepts is actually
the cause of the positive values therein attained. In this way, evil
is "rhetorically transformed" into the cause of good and a good
in itself.

The fact that all injustice is perpetrated for the sake of attaining other values explains why those who do evil frequently fail to see themselves as acting unjustly. Concerned to excuse and justify their actions (thereby relieving the disintegrative effect of an accusing conscience), they see only the positive values they are seeking to attain and for whose sake they do such harm. Hence we find the strange anomaly that sinners regard themselves as relatively upright persons while saints, who are concerned not to justify themselves before an accusing conscience but to measure themselves against perfect justice, often feel themselves to be great malefactors.

When we consider such acts as abortion or capital punishment or the termination of the lives of the hopelessly ill, it is a pathological concern for self-justification that makes us insensitive to the degree to which these acts violate the sanctity of life. This self-justification is pathological because it aims to excuse and reinforce the will of men for their private happiness rather than exposing human action to the requirements of perfect justice. The effect of self-justification, therefore, is to close men off from the very things that makes possible moral growth.

The only way we can be delivered from this pathological condition is to measure our acts against perfect justice, whether or not we can actually accomplish what such perfection requires. Perfect justice aims, as we have seen, at the simultaneous co-affirmation and co-actualization of happiness, freedom, and reverence for the sanctity of life. It is not perfect justice, therefore, when one person feels he must sacrifice another because of interference with the former's own happiness or freedom. Rather, we can have perfect justice only when one person feels his happiness is identical with the maximization of the happiness, freedom, and the life of others.

Happiness, freedom, and the reverence of life can coincide only if our fellow feeling is expanded to include all life. When this expansion occurs, our self is no longer to be diagrammed as a point within a circle that gradually shades off towards something of which it has no part. The self might now be diagrammed as a centerless area of infinite extent and of equal intensity throughout. The self now includes all beings and it cares equally about each and all. The "expanded self" with its infinitely expanded fellow feelings is, of course, something mystical and spiritual, for the spiritual man no longer identifies himself with his body, his flesh, his blood, and his five senses. Now he feels as close to those who are far away and whom he has never met as he does to those whom he sees and hears daily. Every living being is *already* felt to be his friend, his brother. He knows no strangers. When he sees a new face or hears a voice for the first time, he exclaims in his soul "At last!"

Filled with this spirit which is the unity of all life, a man's greatest happiness can be care (agape). Because there can be an identity between his personal happiness and his seeking and delighting in the happiness of others, he is able to act in a perfectly just way by simultaneously affirming every value of life. The act of the spiritual man is peaceful for he himself is filled with peace. Peace is the greatest of the virtues and values of life since, as we have seen, it alone makes both justice and care (agape) possible. We should add, therefore, to the list of values: (5) *the value of peace* (including the instrumentalities of spiritualization).

EVOLUTION OF VALUES

The five values discriminated above are not "natural" in the sense that one could examine any society and find them all differentiated as they have been in this essay. Rather, I suggest that the discrimination of values presented here presupposes the historical evolution of several stages of human culture. For example, classical Greek ethical reflection focused on the value of happiness and its attainment. It did not know the value of freedom precisely because it had no experience of genuine autonomy. Within classical culture, therefore, slavery was not regarded as an ethical problem.

The European discovery of human freedom, i.e., that the will can legislate values by itself when it adheres strictly to the demands of reason, gave man power over his appetites and established a new basis for ethics. Once this freedom was experienced, the prerequisite of every moral action was then seen to be that it conform to the rule of autonomy. It was in European Christianity that freedom emerged. The struggle to reconcile this value with happiness (and with the classical ethical tradition) has set the problematic of European moral reflection to this day. This concern still animates contemporary academic ethics on both sides of the Atlantic (i.e., the teleological/deontological debate).

In the United States, there was still another ethical development: the discrimination of justice as a pragmatic value-optimizing and harmonizing procedure. This constructive or pragmatic justice is distinct from mere right reason in two respects. (In the European tradition justice and reason/freedom were inseparable.) First, American society allocated a sphere of life to freedom alone. In this sphere persons were said to have "rights" and justice could not intrude upon these rights, but only seek from outside to harmonize the choices of men. Second, American society increasingly harnessed theoretical reason and elective freedom to serve man's constructive visions. Rather than accepting situations and asking what is right (what should a free rational being choose), Americans increasingly sought to construct new kinds of situations in which more things could be right.

The particular scheme of values presented in this essay suggests, therefore, a social evolution. For example, only one who has experienced the distinction between justice and rights can make sense out of it. And one experiences such a distinction only in societies that operate in terms of it, that is, in cultures that are more highly differentiated and evolved. In such cultures persons learn and internalize such value discriminations in the course of their education and social experience. This is why the American youth who boldly protests police brutality as a violation of his rights is, I suggest, more developed morally *in this respect* than even Socrates in his cell.

By discriminating among several values, therefore, I am hoping to explain why within the evolution of human morality a new value orientation is emerging. It is an orientation towards peace and spiritualization. Considerations that reflect this new orientation must increasingly influence our experience of and arguments from freedom and justice. And peace must increasingly become the central category in terms of which we rethink all ethical questions. From this new perspective, therefore, abortion is seen to be a morally insensitive act.

However, I know many persons who read this essay will not find its argument persuasive. *This is because they know that in the biological sphere of life women have not yet experienced genuine freedom.* In the past, woman's sexuality has been discussed almost exclusively in terms of happiness. Through motherhood she has been said to fulfill her nature and find satisfaction. For her to refuse motherhood, at any point, has been called "unnatural." Refusal of motherhood has not been interpreted until very recently as woman's gaining freedom over the biological dimensions of her life. It is because the question of abortion is for the first time being articulated in terms of the value of freedom — of woman's right to control her own body, of her freedom to decide whether or not to bear a child — that the desire for abortion law reform can be regarded as a moral step forward. This does not mean that the action of abortion itself must be judged morally right. It means only that a person's demand to decide for himself whether he will nor will not do what is right is an evidence of moral maturation. It is never good for a person to do something that violates perfect justice. But at a certain stage in human moral development it is actually more unjust to require people (through the institution of law) to choose the thing that perfect justice requires than to permit people (through the removal of law) to reject it.

We must be clear about this point: that the legal prohibition of abortion is *relatively unjust* because it sacrifices the value of freedom to the value of reverence for life. Opponents of abortion law reform tend to be insensitive to *this* injustice. On the other hand, an abortion freely chosen (whether in defiance of existing law or in consequence of its abolition) is relatively unjust because it affirms the value of freedom while denying the value of reverence for life.

In this situation, therefore, we must choose between two relatively unjust solutions. Our choice must not be the cynical one that denies the relevance of perfect justice, but must be one that leaves open and affirms the possibility of *further moral growth* toward it.

With these considerations in mind, it would seem that the best solution to the abortion dilemma in the United States is the removal of all laws proscribing it. Such a solution is not perfectly just, but it maximizes the largest number of human values and offers a better way to regulate this matter, i.e., by allowing the persons involved to regulate themselves.

The strongest impediment to the attainment of such personal responsibility, in the present situation, is the very abortion laws that prohibit persons from accepting it. This does not mean, of course, that abortions *will decrease* immediately following the removal of such laws. Quite the contrary is to be expected. This is because personal freedom, limited by a threatening law, can only keep itself alive by imaginations of disobedience and through threats of rebellion. The removal of law may well lead to the actual doing of that which was imagined and threatened beforehand.

Even if this occurs, however, the situation is relatively as just as one that eliminates both abortion and freedom together. This is because the elimination of abortion laws is not simply for the sake of affirming the value of freedom, but also because the attainment of freedom is the "next step" in persons growing toward more perfect justice. At present, the laws bar the way to this maturation.

Those who have lived only under the law cannot believe that persons would freely choose the good that the law prescribes *after that law* has been removed. They depend on something outside themselves to compensate for a moral deficiency within themselves. By now we have had enough experience in dealing with other social problems to know how deficient is the psychology that legalistic morality supposes to be "normal." Free persons, following the first moments of excess and disorientation once the law is removed, then begin voluntarily to do what is good.

8. THE SANCTITY OF LIFE

by Daniel Callahan

O NE PRICE of progress is the substitution of new problems for old. That mankind seems willing enough to pay it does not make the new problems any the less real, or fearsome. The advances of medicine, technology and the life sciences have meant, among other things, a lowering of infant mortality rates, the gradual conquest of disease and disabilities, a longer life expectancy and the possibility of family limitation and population control. One can legitimately call that "progress"; mankind has indeed won for itself the possibility of greater physical security. Yet in many instances these same advances have put before man new moral dilemmas or altered the character of some old ones.

If one were seeking the most characteristic mark of these dilemmas, it might well be located in the rapid expansion of the range of human alternatives. Yet the greater the number of alternatives, the greater the number of difficult choices which must be made; the greater the number of choices, the greater the possibility of confusion, disagreement, and poor judgment. On minor issues, this concatenation of possibilities may be a source of delight and the chance of poor judgment inconsequential. On major issues, however, one may — and should — tremble. The choices will make a difference, to ourselves and to others; any delight that choices *can* be made should be tempered by the sobering thought that they increasingly *must* be made.

The issue of human control over life and death is crucial. What are the responsibilities of those doctors charged with selecting critically ill patients for treatment with artificial kidney machines? There are very few of these machines and very few specialists capable of using them, but there are many people who will surely die if denied such treatment. (The National Kidney Foundation estimates that 5,000–10,000 people die from kidney conditions each year, many of whom could be saved.) Who should be chosen to live and who, unselected, allowed to die? The possibility of a heart transplant is thrilling, but even with better techniques, there are unlikely to be enough heart surgeons in the foreseeable future to take care of all those whose lives could be thus saved. And how are these expensive operations to be paid for (so far, they have cost from $25,000 to $50,000)? Where, in any event, are the hearts to come from – from the "dying" or "dead"? But how can we be sure that someone is "dying" or "dead"? What do we mean by those words? If a person's respiration, circulation, and heart activity are kept going by artificial means, but his brain has ceased functioning, is he "dead"?. This question will be of interest not only to the doctor looking for a sound heart for transplant purposes, but even more frequently by those doctors and families who, in other circumstances, must decide whether to cease artificial support of incurably ill, unconscious patients. What are the obligations of the doctor, of the family, of the hospital, of society? It may soon be possible to engineer genetically the future of human families and, beyond that, the future of the human species. Should this be done? If so, by whom and under what conditions? Experiments with animals and humans have shown the possibility of chemically and electrically altering human emotions and consciousness. How far can we go with such treatment? Medical science depends upon experimentation with human subjects. What are the moral conditions and limits of such work?

These are only some of the pressing questions. There are many more, and each one raises a complex set of sub-questions. And like so many contemporary moral queries, any attempted answers compel us to face in broad terms the human use of technological power, the relationship between moral principles and technical data, the difficulties in achieving workable definitions and consensuses, the place of law and authority. How can we even begin to sort all of these complexities?

One tempting solution must be limited from the start: the

flat rule that since ours is a pluralistic society, every man should be left free to work out these questions for himself and live with his own answers. No doubt there are many circumstances in which this kind of solution would be workable enough, and there is much in the western tradition to commend it as a general moral course. Unhappily, though, the nature of modern society and technology poses some serious obstacles to purely private solutions, and the nature of many of the problems themselves pose others.

On the social plane, the proliferation of state supported hospitals and research facilities very often means that people come together only in relatively impersonal, professional relationships. At times, the layman, whether as client or patient or experiment subject, is wholly at the mercy of a professional or an institution. The possibilities of abuse here are considerable, perhaps less because of any deliberate attempt to misuse professional or institutional power than due to the indifference and insensitivity which impersonal, fleeting relationships often carry with them, particularly when large masses of people are handled or treated. The very proliferation of specialists who can intervene in the life process is staggering: neurosurgeons, geneticists, psychiatrists, and pharmacologists, to mention a few. More people than ever before are involved. It is crucially important, therefore, that there be some publicly acknowledged and respected norms. Professional codes provide one check and public laws still another. But beyond these necessary safeguards, there should also exist, below the surface, something approximating a moral and professional consensus. There are always, for the clever, ways of circumventing codes and laws; a moral consensus is needed to help minimize these circumventions.

The existence of trust and a framework for mutual understanding are critical here. When people put their lives or their bodies in the hands of others, they must be able to do so with reasonable security. In a massive, complicated society, it is not always possible for people to pick their own doctors, to choose those they can rely on. They need the security of knowing that even those doctors, technicians and researchers they meet only in impersonal circumstances will abide by rules and practices common to their profession. On a personal level, it is an unpleasant fact that human beings have been known to kill each other, manipulate each other, and use each other for self-interested ends. No way has yet been devised which completely stops this sort of thing, but the existence of a moral consensus, backed by adequate laws and codes, is some help. Again, trust is necessary: that others will not, by and large, lie to us, try to misuse us, or try to manipulate us. Up to a point, a plurality of moral perspectives is a source of creative tension, producing personal freedom. Beyond that point, often indeterminate, agreement and consensus are necessary, especially when the life of one person is in the hands of another. The destruction of the Jews by the Nazis was not a tribute to the creative power of different moral perspectives.

The obstacles to a moral pluralism posed on the level of the medical and technical problems themselves are no less considerable. Most of the important questions of life and death involve a multiplicity of human relationships. An unconscious patient in the hands of a doctor, an experimental subject under the control of a researcher, and a future mutation of the human species in the hands of a small group of geneticists are all circumstances where one person or one group is in the position of making choices which affect others.

If, then, some minimal degree of moral consensus is necessary on matters of life and death, what is it and on what can it be based? Without some fundamental points of moral agreement, laws cannot be framed, codes enacted, or trust engendered. To a certain degree, sensible men can enact statutes which reflect only a pragmatic agreement to abide by certain rules. But even an apparently pragmatic agreement on sheerly procedural questions will almost always reflect some latent value commitment, viz., that it is good that procedures for settling disputes among men exist. Fortunately, in the principle of "the sanctity of life," western culture (and much of eastern culture as well) possesses one fundamental basis for an approach to moral consensus; that is, we are not forced to begin from within a sheer vacuum. On the basis of this principle, moral rules have been framed, human rights claimed and defended, and cultural, political, and social priorities established.

To be sure, the principle is vague in its wording, erratically affirmed in practice, and open to innumerable differences in interpretation. (For instance, Werner Schöllgen and Joseph Fletcher express distaste for the phrase because they believe it implies a crude vitalism, exalting life as such, whatever its quality [24:217; 11:62]. But I do not feel common usage gives it this connotation.) The word "sanctity," for example, carries a religious connotation not always congenial to the non-religious. "Life" does not clearly specify whether all life (as in the Hindu version) or only human life is meant. Nonetheless, the frequency of the use of the principle in ethical discussions, even by the non-religious, testifies to its continuing utility, at least as a point of departure. In any case, there seems to be no other widely affirmed principle which presently serves as well. Perhaps a better formulation for the thrust of this principle could be found — for instance, "the dignity of human life." But if one's aim is moral consensus, then it is wise to seek not originality of formulation, however brilliant, but as common and widely understood a principle as possible, one which still lives, is still affirmed, and still has deep cultural resonance.

If "the sanctity of life" is, preeminently, our basic western principle, what does it mean, where has it come from, and how can it effectively be utilized in moral decisions and the formation of moral consensus? The overall purpose of this paper is to uncover possible grounds for just such a moral consensus, and, though I will concern myself with some substantive matters, the paper is primarily structural in aim. The first task is to clarify the meaning of "the sanctity of life"; this can usefully be done by analyzing some current explanations of it.

THE CHRISTIAN UNDERSTANDING OF "THE SANCTITY OF LIFE"

Paul Ramsey has effectively detailed a major Christian tradition on the origin of the principle of "the sanctity of life." In a discussion of abortion, he observes that "one grasps the religious outlook upon the sanctity of human life only if he sees that this life is asserted to be *surrounded* by sanctity that need not be in a man; that the most dignity a man ever possesses is a dignity that is alien to him. . . . A man's dignity is an overflow from God's dealing with him, and not primarily an anticipation of anything he will ever be by himself alone" [21:71]. Prof. Ramsey goes on to say that "The value of a human life is ultimately grounded in the value God is placing on it," and his point here is twofold [21:72]. First, it is to make clear that in the religious view, the sanctity of human life is not a function of the worth any human being may attribute to it; this therefore precludes discussion of any "degrees of relative worth" a human being may have or acquire. "Life's primary value," stemming from God, transcends such distinctions. Second, Ramsey wants to make clear that a man's life "is entirely an ordination, a loan, and a stewardship. His essence is his existence before God and to God, and it is from Him" [21:73]. In this formulation, man must respect his own life and the life of others not only because it is grounded in God, but, equally important, because God has given man life as a value to be held in trust and used according to God's will. "Respect for life," Ramsey writes, "does not mean that a man must live and let live from some iron law of necessity, or even that there is a rational compulsion to do this, or a rational ground for doing so. It is rather that because God has said 'Yes' to life, man's 'yes' should echo His" [21:76]. Ramsey adds that it is not terribly important which specific Christian doctrine one emphasizes to reach this conclusion; any number point in the same direction, whether it be the doctrine of creation, of man's creation in the image of God, of God's covenantal relationship with His people, or the doctrine of Redemption [21:74].

Like other Protestant theologians, Ramsey makes prominent use of Karl Barth's theology of creation. In emphasizing the "respect" due human life, Barth wants to give the word "respect" a deep resonance, indicating that we should stand in awe of that human life which God has granted man: "Respect is man's astonishment, humility and awe at a fact in which he meets something superior — majesty, dignity, holiness, a mystery which compels him to withdraw and keep his distance, to handle it modestly, circumspectly and carefully. . . . In human life he meets something superior" [3]. Martin J. Buss and Helmut Thielicke have argued similarly to Ramsey and Barth. Thielicke, in particular, stresses that a theory of "alien dignity" protects human life from being subjected to utilitarian treatment at the hands of other human beings; the measure of human value is not man's "functional proficiency" or "pragmatic utility," but rather "the sacrificial love which God has invested in him" [27:231]. In Buss' words, "Theologically . . . the worth of man lies in his being addressed by a deity" [7:249].

On the whole, the traditional Catholic analyses of the origin of life closely parallel the Protestant, emphasizing God as the source and ultimate guarantor of the sanctity of human life. Thus Josef Fuchs, S.J., asserts that "man as such belongs *directly and exclusively to God*" [12:65]. Norman St. John-Stevas, who has written more extensively on "the sanctity of life" than any other recent Roman Catholic, has said that "Respect for the *lives* of others because of their eternal destiny is the essence of the Christian teaching. Its other aspect is the emphasis on the creatureliness of man. Man is not absolutely master of his own life and body. He has no *dominium* over it, but holds it in trust for God's purposes" [23:12]. This emphasis on God's purposes, man's creatureliness and man's holding of life in trust brings the Catholic and Protestant arguments together at a critical point. Catholic theories, however, have been much more likely than Protestant ones to stress, through man's discernment of the natural law apart from revelation, the ability of reason to ascertain the source of the sanctity of life. Quite apart from an acceptance of Christian revelation, man, according to Catholic natural law arguments, should be able to recognize man's dignity. As G. Kelly has put it, "only God has the right to take the life of the innocent; hence the direct killing of the innocent, without the authority of God, is always wrong. This truth we know through human nature (natural law) and through divine revelation (the divine positive law) . . ." [18:165]. But even Father Kelly, having asserted that we can understand the sanctity of life and the right to life through the natural law, concedes that it is not altogether easy to prove the point through reason alone: "The reason for this difficulty seems to be that to those who really believe in creation and the supreme dominion of God, the principle is too obvious to need proof; whereas for those who do not believe in creation there is no basis on which to build a proof" [18:167].

In any event, Catholic thought as much as Protestant has pushed the sanctity of life back to a divine origin and preservation, to an "alien dignity" (though most Catholic theologians would not find that phrase very congenial because of its suggestion that man's rights are not inherent). Within this basic perspective, however, some nuances are frequently added, mainly of a pragmatic nature. St. John-Stevas adds to his argument that the sanctity of life stems from God the further contentions (a) that it is a fundamental principle which has sustained western society, the rejection or dilution of which would endanger the whole of human life and (b) that in any case, there is no other principle available which would provide a "criterion of the right to life, save that of personal taste" [23:17]. His fully rounded argument for the sanctity of life draws, finally, on many sources: western law and history, human experience, the Christian doctrine of man, and the continuing cultural necessity that such a principle be accepted [22:46].

Central to both Catholic and Protestant theology is the principle that God is the Lord of life and death [16:194; 8:27]. This is another way of proclaiming that man holds his own life in trust, another way of asserting that man's ultimate value stems from God, and another way of saying that no man can take it upon himself to place himself in total mastery over the life of another. To confess that God is lord of life and death is to affirm that man is a creature, owing his existence, his value, and his ultimate destiny to God. But like the related principle of the sanctity of life, it is a principle which conceals some difficulties. One of these is the relationship of God to the moral and physical evils of the world. Christian theodicy has long wrestled with the apparently contradictory belief that God is lord and yet that his lordship is not responsible for evil [17]. Another difficulty is that both in principle and practice Christian theology has allowed many occasions when it is permissible for one man to take the life of another, or for the state to take the life, or imprison the body, of those it considers dangerous to the common good. Such exceptions clearly seem to presuppose that in some sense God has granted man some degree of control over human life and death, a presupposition shared by Catholic and Protestant theologians.

As the history of Christian ethics shows, it has never been possible to take decisions out of human hands for long. Even before the advent of modern technology choices had to be made among human lives and human rights. Unjust aggression, for example, raised the question whether God's sanctification of human life was consistent with laws which, in effect, granted aggressors the right to take innocent lives. The historical answer was no; hence were born laws which granted individuals and communities the right to take the lives of aggressors or deprive them of other rights. In other words, it turned out that here, as in many other instances, human decisions had to be made; they could not be left to God. The inherent stability supposedly built into a divine sanctity of life principle turned out to be something less than perfect. The present turmoil of Christian ethics is due precisely to a growing awareness that rigid, formalistic ethical codes too often break down in practice, all the more so because of the expanded range of possible choice.

While it may be perfectly reasonable to suppose that man has been given some proximate control over human life, it is a supposition which also places upon human shoulders the problem of deciding under what conditions man has the right to such control. But once these decisions have to be made, there is the danger that the principle of God's lordship may be emptied of any meaningful content. If it is man who must decide what it means to implement this lordship, of what real good is the abstract principle? This is a question to which I will return.

The advantages of the Christian approach to "the sanctity of life" are evident, just as are some of the disadvantages. The main advantage is that the foundation is laid for a theory of human life which locates man's dignity outside the evaluation of other human beings; our ultimate worth is conferred by God, not by human judgment. Thus, in principle, human life is guaranteed beyond the protection that an erratic human evaluation might accord it, whether in the form of human laws or mores. Another advantage is that the sanctity of human life is given an ultimate grounding: in God, the creator and preserver of everything which exists. Man is not forced to create his own worth; God has, from the outset, given him value.

The disadvantages, however, are no less prominent. One is that a considerable portion of humanity is not Christian and does not accept this foundation for the sanctity of human life. Hence, it does not readily provide a consensual norm to which all men can have recourse. Another disadvantage is that it leaves unclear the extent of man's intrinsic dignity. It seems to presuppose that, apart from God's conferral of dignity, man in his own right would be worthless. In the theological problematic of course, which is all-encompassing in its scope, it makes no sense to talk of man apart from his creator and redeemer; the "natural man" does not exist, but only the created and redeemed man. In part, this helps to solve the problem of an "alien dignity" which would denigrate man's intrinsic worth, but, at the same time, it requires that one accept the full theological framework; that is just what many cannot do. In his *Ethics*, Dietrich Bonhoeffer speaks of a "natural right" to bodily life, thus more consciously than most Protestant theologians trying to establish a continuum between a secular mode of describing human rights and a strictly Christian mode. But even Bonhoeffer, who uses a term such as "innate right," sees the guarantee and source of these rights wholly in God [6:106 ff].

THE EXPERIENTIAL UNDERSTANDING OF "THE SANCTITY OF LIFE"

Very different from the Christian position are the arguments put forward by Edward Shils and P. D. Medawar to justify the sanctity of life. Pointing to what seems an almost instinctive human revulsion at many forms of contrived intervention in human life, Shils believes that it is not possible to trace this revulsion solely to the religious belief that man is a creature of God. On the contrary, he contends that the Christian belief in the sanctity of life has been sustained by a "deeper, protoreligious 'natural metaphysic,'" which also accounts for the respect given human life by those who are neither Christian nor religious [25:9]. "The chief feature of the protoreligious 'natural metaphysic' is the affirmation that life *is* sacred. It is believed to be sacred not because it is a manifestation of a transcendent creator from whom life comes: it is believed to be sacred because it is life. The idea of sacredness is generated by the primordial experience of being alive, of experiencing the elemental sensation of vitality and the elemental fear of its extinction" [25:12]. In another place he writes that "If life were not viewed as sacred, then nothing else would be sacred," thus echoing from within his own framework the same kind of pragmatic point made by Norman St. John-Stevas from within a very different kind of framework [25:14–15]. Finally, Shils says: "The question still remains: is human life really sacred? I answer that it is, self-evidently. Its sacredness is the most primordial of experiences" [25:18].

Like the Christian formulation of the principle, Shils' way of putting the matter has both strengths and weaknesses. Its obvious strength is that the sanctity of human life does not require a justification outside of human life (i.e., in a God), thus providing a basis upon which the non-religious can affirm the sanctity of life, something which the Christian formulation does not. It also has the advantage of drawing directly upon human experience, and very root human experience at that; no divine revelation is required. Its chief weakness is that it falls afoul of some obvious philosophical rejoinders. The first would be that the mere experiencing of something as valuable is no guarantee that it *is* valuable. People frequently experience something as valuable which later reflection shows to be lacking in value, and it is common for different groups of people to experience different things as valuable. The second rejoinder would be that Shils' case could not be fully established unless we had evidence that all human beings have at all times experienced human life as valuable; it is not easy to see how this could be done. The third rejoinder would be that "the sanctity of human life" is a human concept, one which has been considered appropriate to ascribe to certain elemental human experiences. But this ascription already presupposes the existence of a conceptual and linguistic system which may be utilized in describing experience; such a utilization, though, requires making judgments about experience, particularly judging that certain experiences are valuable. But what we decide to call a "value" will be a function of prior ethical decisions. On all three of these points, Shils' phrase "self-evidently" quoted above opens the way to a host of objections. P. B. Medawar, whose defense of the sanctity of life is similar to but more sketchy than that of Shils, rests his case upon "a certain natural sense of the fitness of things, a feeling that is shared by most kind and reasonable people even if we cannot define it in philosophically defensible or legally accountable terms" [20:98]. The same kinds of objections could be leveled at this argument as have been suggested against Shils' approach, but perhaps even more strongly: it is notorious, for example, that different people and different cultures have very different senses of "the fitness of things"; it is a norm which does not provide very reliable criteria in judging the nature of things.

AN IMPASSE

Now if both the Christian understanding of "the sanctity of life" and the experiential, non-religious interpretation put foward by Shils and Medawar are open to internal objections, each also provides the grounds for a critique of the other. One important intent of the Christian understanding is to remove the ultimate source of the sanctity of life from any dependence upon human experience and judgment; this is accomplished by locating the source of the sanctity outside man. Extending Shils' argument, though, could not one say that the precise weakness of this kind of extrinsic grounding is that it requires one to affirm not only human sanctity but the source of that sanctity as well? Two affirmations are necessary, making it doubly difficult to make *any* affirmation. Moreover, it could be said that an acceptance of the sanctity of life which required that one accept a religious view of man's origin would provide a weak base upon which to build a consensus; one then would seem to be saying that there would be nothing upon which to base the sanctity of life save that of religious belief (which would logically leave the non-believer free to reject the sanctity of life). One untoward consequence, then, of the religious believer's position would be to open the way to placing his own right to life in jeopardy, by making the sanctity of his own life dependent only upon his own religious beliefs. Beyond his own beliefs, he would have nothing to appeal to in the face of aggressive action by a person denying these beliefs. An intrinsic norm for the sanctity of life, such as that proposed by Shils and Medawar, would seem to avoid such untoward consequences. For it would, in principle, provide a norm to which all men could have recourse (or could have pointed out to them); one would need only to refer to a (purportedly) universal human experience and not be dependent upon any special belief about the nature of man and the source of his dignity.

At this point, however, the religious believer could point out how precarious such an intrinsic norm is. To be an effective norm, it would first have to be shown that all men are in fact, or potentially, aware of such an elemental experience of the sanctity of life. It would further have to be shown that human beings have a moral obligation to heed this experience, that the experience carries with it a manifest set of moral obligations. The fact that I might respect the sanctity of my own life, my own vitality, does not logically entail that I am required to respect the sanctity of anyone else's life. What would be the source of any obligation to respect the life of another? The mere existence of a common human experience would, on the face of it, entail no moral obligations or duties at all. Only the experience of an ethical framework superimposed upon the experience could supply these entailments. The strength of the believer's extrinsic norm is that it bypasses these difficulties; it is not dependent upon any particular human experience, it does not have to work through the hazardous business of proving that moral duties are inherent in human experience, and it provides an ethical framework binding upon all in principle. At this point, though, all the difficulties inherent in the believer's position recur. We are at an impasse.

Now it is surely conceivable that some ingenious person could find a way out of this impasse — conceivable, but not likely — at least not likely in the sense that his way out would commend itself to all sides in the debate. The very nature of the debate, which in the end opposes two fundamentally different world-views, precludes the likelihood of a common theoretical solution, short of the conversion of one side or the other. In one sense, then, we seem to be in the presence of an ill-fated debate, one which appears doomed to go on forever, perennially resistant to the formation of a socially useful moral consensus, perennially prone to leave the principle of the sanctity of life in a dangerous position. I don't think it is necessary to draw this kind of pessimistic conclusion. For one thing, it is always difficult to metaphysically ground first, or ultimate, principles but this difficulty does not necessarily stand in the way of their acceptance and use. In social, political, cultural, and medical situations, what counts most in the debate on the sanctity of life is that both sides affirm the principle, on whatever grounds, and that both sides are willing to make it their first and fundamental principle. Moreover, it is clear from a variety of human disciplines that their practitioners can often effectively talk and work together without metaphysical agreement on fundamental principles, or even when the fundamental principles themselves carry no evident intrinsic justification. The problem of induction in the philosophy of science provides a classic instance. Scientific method presupposes that the future will be like the past, that hypotheses confirmed by observed data provide a warrant for making predictions about similar, but unobserved, data, that it is legitimate to base expectations about the future behavior of material objects on our present experience with such objects. Yet it has proved exceedingly difficult to demonstrate the philosophical validity of these presuppositions [see 2]. Nonetheless, the enterprise of science has been able to proceed and progress in the absence of such demonstrations and in the absence of a full philosophical consensus on the ultimate validity of scientific method.

Another way of expressing this general point is by observing that no method or first principle is self-justifying; it is always logically permissible to ask that a methodology be justified in terms other than its own, just as it is equally permissible to ask for a justification of the justification ad infinitum of a first principle. For all that, by affirming the utility of certain methods and the value of certain first principles human beings have effectively developed themselves, their knowledge, and their behavior. Both Norman St. John-Stevas and Edward Shils, though differing on the source of the sanctity of life, agree on its value as a first principle, and both make use of a similar collateral pragmatic argument. "If life were not viewed and experienced as sacred, then nothing else would be sacred," Shils writes [25:14–15]. "Once exceptions are made [to the principle of the sanctity of life], the whole structure of human rights is undermined," is the way St. John-Stevas puts it [23:14]. Both are saying, in effect, the same thing: if you want to make anything sacred, if you want any values honored, if you want to be able to defend any rights, then it is necessary to postulate the principle of the sanctity of life (or presumably, a principle with the same general thrust). There is of course a long philosophical debate behind the validity of arguments taking this logical form (especially from Kant forward); suffice it to say that, if one's concern is to make use of an available ground of practical consensus, effective consensuses have been built on a common acceptance of arguments taking this logical form.

But a further, and critical, problem arises. Even if there is agreement that "the sanctity of human life" is worth affirming, indeed socially imperative to affirm, it appears to be singularly abstract and ambiguous as a principle. If it is possible to derive from this principle a huge variety of often divergent moral rules and duties, simply because it is open to human beings to interpret the principle in different ways, and if, in practice, the widespread affirmation of the principle does not lead to any unified consensus on what it implies, and if each of the important words in the principle — "sanctity," "human," and "life" — is itself open to different and divergent definitions — then of what conceivable value is such a principle? Are we not perhaps deluding ourselves in trying to hold on to the principle, or in thinking that it can serve as a basis for consensus? Doesn't it just raise more problems than it solves?

"THE SANCTITY OF LIFE" AS AN ABSTRACT PRINCIPLE

In "Levels of Moral Discourse," Henry D. Aiken has provided a perceptive justification of the value and utility of an abstract principle of this kind [1:65 – 87]. Aiken distinguishes four "levels" of moral discourse: an expressive-evocative, a moral, an ethical, and a post-ethical level. At the expressive-evocative level, people simply express their personal feelings: "ugh," "hurray," "good!" They are expressed in such a way that "They do not solicit agreement or invite a reply" [1:69]. The "moral" level is where "serious questions are asked and serious answers given . . . 'What ought I to do in this situation?' 'Is this object that I admire so much, really good?' . . . Here, in short, there now appears a problem of conduct and a problem for appraisal and ultimate decision" [1:70]. What is characteristic, however, of our reasoning at the moral level is that we normally operate within the given rules or codes of our community (social, religious, or ideological), trying to apply these accepted rules to concrete situations. Yet if this is what people normally do, "Occasionally one is obliged to ask whether an action which is prescribed by existing moral rules *really* is right and whether, therefore, one ought to continue to obey them. When pressed in a certain way, the effect of such a question is to throw doubt upon the validity of the rules themselves. And in that case, there is usually no alternative to a fundamental reconsideration of the whole moral code" [1:75].

It is when we are faced with this alternative that we are forced to move to still another level of moral discourse, what Aiken calls the "ethical" level. It is at this level that very general, very abstract, and very formal principles (e.g., "the sanctity of life") show their value. It is the function of such principles to place practical questions arising from our use of a rule system "on a level of impersonality which requires the subordination of personal bias or preference. It is their function to establish a mood in which the particular moral rule or the moral code as a whole is considered impartially . . . . without regard to our own inclinations or benefits. . . . A second characteristic effect of this use of ethical terms is their tendency to 'frame' or set apart the questions and answers in which they occur from ordinary practical deliberations" [1:76].

Aiken's response to the objection that ethical principles are "empty" because of their vagueness — and that is a major objection to the principle of "the sanctity of life" — is to point out that their function is "procedural rather than substantive in aim. Their role is not to tell us what to do in particular cases (the function of a moral rule system) but to provide us with standards of relevance or 'reasonableness' when appraisal of lower order rules is required"[1:82]. In order to perform this kind of function the principle must be "empty," must be formal. To give it a specific content would be to turn it into a rule; what we need, when we want to test or validate a rule, is not another rule (which could lead to an infinite succession of rules), but a principle for judging all our rules. An "ethical" principle is "not a rule of conduct but a formula for testing rules of conduct. . . . To enrich its content would be *ipso facto* to transform its role and hence to deprive it of its power as a general principle of ethical criticism" [1:82].

As we have seen, both Shils and St. John-Stevas agree on the need for the principle of the sanctity of life, even though they totally disagree on its source. Now we can see exemplified in their justification of the need a point Aiken makes about Kant's defense of "empty," high level ethical principles: "What he [Kant] saw with unrivaled clarity, is that moral criticism which is something more than an *ad hoc* expression of individual attitudes is impossible save on the assumption that there are ethical principles which are general in normative appeal" [1:82]. When Shils and St. John-Stevas say that no human rights and no valuation of human life can be established without presupposing "the sanctity of life" they are saying no less than what Kant said.

Put more concretely, it is possible to see the function of the principle of the sanctity of life. If one asks, for example, "Is it a good general rule that abortions ought not to be performed?" — to take a rule which has until recently been a part of the western moral rule system — one needs a principle which operates at a higher level than the particular rule in order to judge the validity of the rule. "The sanctity of life" provides such a principle. Does that particular rule about abortion serve or enhance or exemplify "the sanctity of life"? That is the kind of question we will want to ask about the rule. That is the kind of question the principle is meant to help us answer; it provides a way of testing the rule, giving us a "frame" within which to validate it anew or to invalidate or amend it.

One might object that the principle could not serve as a measure or test of a particular rule if it was, quite literally and totally, empty. Here I think Aiken's account of the function of general ethical principles needs some correction. Instead of saying that these principles are "empty," it might be preferable to say that they are "indeterminate" — they convey a broad range of meaning, but not specific, determinate meanings. We know what the principle is trying to express — roughly. We know what the principle would seem to preclude — vaguely. We know, consequently, how to use the principle as a measure of rules — more or less. If asked to specify what the phrase "the sanctity of life" *means*, we could substitute phrases like "the dignity," "the ultimate value," "the worth," "the significance," "the importance" of human life for the phrase "the sanctity" — trying, all the while, to hit upon that phrase or combination of phrases which would make clear what we had in mind when we spoke of the principle or what we take to be the principle, as commonly used, to mean. Naturally, someone could point out that defining the words of the principle in terms of a list of synonyms or near-synonyms is not altogether illuminating, having about it the odor of tautologies and circularities. About the only thing one could reply, if faced with this kind of resistance, is that one reaches a point, with any word or any phrase or any ultimate principle, where one simply cannot say anything more. The point about the phrase "the sanctity of life" is that it is trying to say the *most* that can be said about the value of life. It signifies a whole cluster of final meanings, each of which is related to and dependent upon the other to give it sense and significance. In a very real way, then, the principle of the sanctity of life *is* indeterminate and vague, but not meaningless for all that. It says life is to be affirmed, cherished, and respected, and as a principle, it can be defined in terms of a large range of words which themselves have meaning, yet without this process of definition overdefining the principle (which would make it too determinate to be useful as an ethical principle). When used in its primary function of judging lower level rules, the principle is employed to interrogate the rules: do the rules foster the respect due human life? Do the rules lead people to protect human life? Do the rules exemplify the awe we ought to feel in the presence of human life? If the answer is "no," then we would be justified in rejecting, modifying or changing the rules.

Yet further specificity is required here. If it is the general function of moral rules to guide our conduct in particular situations calling for moral decisions — "What ought I to do?" — there is also a multiplicity of rules and a multiplicity of ways in which rules are expressed. The reason for a multiplicity of rules is not hard to locate: there are many different kinds of human acts, human relationships, and human moral dilemmas. Sometimes we are concerned with human property, at other times with human lives, at other times with human political rights, at other times with human sexual duties, at other times with human economic relationships. Different general contexts call for and ordinarily exhibit different sets of rules, even though there may be and usually is a considerable overlap. The reason for a multiplicity of ways in which to express rules can be readily seen also. Sometimes rules are expressed in the form of prohibitions — "Thou shalt not. . . ." This form of rule statement is meant to draw a line beyond which one may not go; prohibitions set limits. Sometimes rules are expressed in a positive way — "One ought to do 'x,'" "One must do 'y'" — and the aim here is to specify a duty or a responsibility; a goal is established. In brief, rules are variously expressed in the language of rights, duties, prohibitions, goals, and so on, and these different expressions have different purposes: to command, to enjoin, to goad, and so on. And it is usually possible to translate one mode of expressing a rule into another mode: the prohibition "Thou shalt not steal" can be re-expressed into the command "You ought to respect the property of others," though the psychological impact of the re-expression may be somewhat different from the original expression, and the implications for behavior rather different.

The important point is to understand the possible ways that the ethical principle of "the sanctity of life" can be used to test those moral rules bearing on human life. We have already seen that the *meaning* of "the sanctity of life" is that of signifying the ultimate respect we are willing to accord human life. It expresses a willingness to treat human life with consideration, to give it dignity, to commit ourselves to its furtherance. The function of specific rules is to implement and give concreteness to these commitments; in turn these commitments, as summed up in the principle, will serve to judge the adequacy of the rules. Thus the relationship between particular moral rules and general ethical principles is reciprocal: the rules give content, on a lower level, to the principle; the principle, on a higher level, is used to judge the rules. The social importance of the acceptance of the principle of "the sanctity of life" is not that it guarantees agreement on what the rules should be, or that recourse to it automatically resolves disputes about rules, but that a common standard exists which people can have recourse to; debate about rules has a framework of meaning, vague though it may be.

Another point is important here. When, as will be shown, we break the different rule systems down into relevant categories, it is helpful to see the way in which the different categories are related to each other. The greater the degree of relationship we can see among the categories, the more we are illuminated about, and in a position to give meaning to, "the sanctity of life." This is another way the principle provides a framework for discussing rules and rule systems. It leads us to see, it can even force us to see, that when dealing with the complexity of human life our rules should have a coherent relationship to each other. It leads us to see, to express the point another way, that *our rules should form a coherent system, each rule consistent with and supporting the other*, and all, in turn, serving and supporting the ultimate principle of "the sanctity of life." Rules dealing with medical experimentation should be congruent with rules dealing with the preservation of an individual's bodily life, which should be congruent with rules dealing with the preservation of the species, and so on. This is simply to say that just as moral rules should not be *ad hoc*, unrelated to an overarching ethical principle, neither should they be *ad hoc* in the sense of being unrelated to other rules bearing on the same overarching ethical principle. To use an image: if the ethical principle is the father of the family, then all the children (the concrete rules) should bear a family resemblance to each other.

When we look more closely at those rules and rule systems bearing on the sanctity of life their variety is manifest. There are rules dealing with (a) the survival and integrity of the human species, (b) the integrity of family lineages, (c) the integrity of bodily life, (d) the integrity of personal, mental, and emotional individuality, and (e) the integrity of personal bodily individuality [suggested by 25:29]. Not one of these areas has escaped the impact of recent medical, scientific, and technological change. It is this change, together with the concomitantly increasing scope of moral decisions, which has brought traditional rules into question and, beyond that, is forcing us to see whether these old rules still serve "the sanctity of life." If not, then new rules will be needed.

A further complication, moreover, is that we will not be in a position to judge the rules in relationship to the guiding principle until we have first determined their relationship to the empirical data to which they are applied. Rules are meant (either explicitly or implicitly) to exemplify principles; but their application must be in the context of data. When the data to which the rules have traditionally been applied change, this can mean either of two things: we will have to judge whether existing rules can handle the new data or whether entirely new rules are needed. Recent debates about the continuing relevance of "just war" theories provide an example of this problem. On one side are those who contend that the advent of nuclear weapons renders the traditional rules of just warfare altogether irrelevant; they were not designed to cope with weapons capable of such vast and indiscriminate destruction. On another side are those who believe that the old rules are sufficiently flexible to handle nuclear warfare. A considerable part of this debate, not surprisingly, turns on an analysis of the known data concerning the destructiveness of nuclear weapons. Short of such an analysis there is no way of knowing whether the traditional rules of just warfare are still valid; and short of knowing that there is no way of judging whether these rules still serve a commitment to the sanctity of life.

THE LEADING RULE SYSTEMS

I now want to survey briefly the leading rule systems subsumed under "the sanctity of life." My aim will be threefold, in line with the major issues I have discussed: to bring out the latent general content of the principle itself, to indicate what appear to be the extant western moral rules, and to point out the kinds of technical data bearing on the individual rule systems, noting in the process the implications of different kinds of data. Since the overall purpose of this paper is to uncover possible grounds for a moral consensus, rather than to propose new rules, I have to risk that my reading of the extant cultural rules is wrong. Obviously different sub-communities within the culture have different rule systems; that is why they argue with each other. And even when they agree on rule systems, they often disagree on the implications of technical data for an application of the rules. Still, I believe it is possible to discern considerable agreement among the different western moral sub-communities, at least if one remains at a fairly high level of abstraction and generality. One test is whether there are any important groups which flatly oppose the cultural rules. In any event, it is open to the reader to supply his own reading of the extant rules in place of mine. The important thing here is to uncover the logical structure of the relationship between rules and the principle of "the sanctity of life," thus laying the basis for fruitful discussion among contending sub-communities.

(a) *The survival and integrity of the human species.* The most important rule here is that the human species ought to work toward its own survival; it is good that human beings exist on earth. Encompassed within this broad rule are a number of other more specific rules: present human beings ought to behave in such a way as to insure as much as possible a viable life for future human beings; nations ought not to behave in such a way as to endanger the present and future life of the human species; human beings are responsible for a moral use of natural resources, and so forth. The rules are myriad and they are invoked, either explicitly or implicitly, when human beings discuss nuclear warfare, radiation exposure, air pollution, ecology, overpopulation, urbanization, the uses of technology, and genetic engineering. The working presumption is that "the sanctity of life" entails the need for moral rules designed to aid the survival of collective human life. Existing rules which can be shown to hinder the possibility of continuing human life would then stand under the judgment of the principle and be subject to rejection or modification.

The problem of genetic engineering, ever expanding in its possibilities, illustrates the complexities of judging old rules and forming new ones. On the one hand, there are questions of technical feasibility. To what extent, and by what means, is it possible to alter the genetic characteristics of human populations? And what are the likely consequences of choosing different means? "Positive eugenics," involving the engineered breeding of a chosen type or types of human being, poses the technical problem of accurately predicting the genetic consequences of different, artificially induced, genetic mixes. "Negative eugenics," generally understood to mean either the discouragement or forbiddance of reproduction by carriers of harmful genes, requires (as does positive eugenics) an ability to predict the long range consequences for human evolution of non-random mating patterns. "Euthenics," the alteration of environment to permit genetically abnormal people to live normal lives, poses the scientific question whether in the long run mankind might become so overburdened with genetic abnormalities as to overwhelm the possibilities of a supporting environmental change. Each of these different possible eugenic techniques, then, requires a knowledge of the different likely genetic outcomes [13]. And any judgment of rules relating to genetic engineering will have to weigh and compare these outcomes.

On the other hand, there are questions concerning the kind of human beings we want now and in the future. Even if one can predict the outcome of different methods of genetic engineering, there still remains the further problem of deciding what characteristics are humanly desirable; and this problem requires some further scientific calculations about the conditions of human life in the future. The rules we judge desirable should, therefore, reflect a scientifically valid use of data combined with a conscious reflection upon the kinds of human beings felt desirable. And of course there is the basic question whether we have the right to do this at all. As a principle, "the sanctity of life" provides no detailed map for wending our way through this maze of problems. But it does tell us this: whatever our evolving moral rules will be, they must be designed to promote the survival of the human species; negatively, the principle tells us that any rule which is oblivious to, or harmful to, the survival of the human species is to be rejected.

(b) *The survival and integrity of family lineages.* The central rule in this instance is that individuals and families should be left free to propagate their own children and to perpetuate their family lineage [cf. 25:22]. Related rules are that neither the state nor other individuals have the right to interfere with private procreative practices; neither the state nor other individuals have the right to impose or deny individual parenthood or to tamper with the process of individual procreation. The intent behind these rules would seem to be that "the sanctity of life" requires respect for family lines and for voluntary procreative choice. Artificial insemination and artificial inovulation, sterilization and contraception, as well as genetic engineering all raise technological options bearing on this rule. Beyond these options are problems concerning the common good of societies and humanity as a whole, the procreative rights of individuals in different circumstances (e.g., in times of overpopulation, or in cases where known and dangerous genetic characteristics would be perpetuated within families or transmitted to a population as a whole). Once again, rules have to be formulated in cognizance of technical knowledge; once again, choices must be made about the kind and number of human beings which families and societies judge desirable.

(c) *The integrity of bodily life.* The general rule in this case is that the individual human being has a basic right to life; neither the state nor individuals have the right to (unjustly) deprive human beings of their lives. This rule encompasses a great range of subsidiary rules, among them rules relating to abortion, euthanasia, the prolongation of moribund life, war, capital punishment, and the like. The presumption behind these rules is that "the sanctity of life" implies not only the preservation of human life as a whole but also the preservation and protection of individual human lives.

As one moves through the different detailed rule systems subsumed under the general rule, a wide range of definitional, technical, and social problems presents itself. Abortion poses the question "When does 'human life' begin?" and that question contains within it the need for a definition of "human life," for criteria which would help us decide what is meant by "begin," and for standards to govern behavior toward potential or incipient human life [see 7:21]. Biological data are relevant to the definition difficulty, the common use of language to the establishment of criteria for "begin," and broad social goals to the forming of standards about potential human life (and these are not the only relevant considerations, just some of them). The prolongation of moribund human life also touches on the definition problem — what do we mean by "death," at what point do we say that, for all practical purposes, a human body ceases being a "human life" [10]? An important technical context of these problems is the possibility of artificially prolonging many bodily functions indefinitely. Euthanasia forces us to ask whether there is a "right to die," and whether, in cases of excruciating pain or a hopeless prognosis we could speak of a "right to kill" even manifestly innocent life. Whatever the continuing or developed rules, however, they would be judged in the light of an accepted implication of "the sanctity of life": human beings have a right to bodily life; any rule which threatens that right is nullified by the principle of the sanctity of life.

(d) *The integrity of personal, mental, and emotional individuality* [4]. The key rule here is that a person has the right to be himself; phrased differently, a human being has the right to be a unique person with his own complement of voluntarily chosen mental and emotional traits (as far as is possible biologically and psychologically). Related rules are that neither the state nor other individuals have the right to tamper with or impair individual human minds or to manipulate, coerce, or alter human emotions. These rules are called into question by the possibility of electrical and chemical alterations of consciousness and affectivity which could well be judged beneficial, either to the individual or society or both. The technical problem here is that of measuring the short and long term effects of such alterations, both on the individual and on a society made up of such individuals. The impact of the use of hallucinogenics is a case in point, as is the existence of brain operations, tranquilizers, drugs, and electrical treatments which can affect thought and emotions. Whatever the rules here, worked out in relationship to scientific knowledge of the effects of different mind- and emotion-altering techniques, they are meant to embody the general rule that a person has the right to be himself. This rule is an implication of the affirmation that "the sanctity of life" entails the value of personal identity.

(e) *The integrity of personal bodily individuality.* The guiding rule in this instance is that the individual has an exclusive right to the use of his own body and all the organs therein; one should respect the integrity of human bodies. This rule comes into question when the need for medical experimentation arises, when organ transplants are required, and when (as in wartime) society may feel it necessary to place the body or bodily life of its citizens in physical jeopardy. The "need for medical experimentation" involves such technical questions as the likely scientific results which could accrue from such experimentations, the relative degree of danger involved in different kinds of experimentation, the scientific value of informing or failing to inform experimental subjects of the purpose of the experimentation (e.g., when a new pain-killing drug is being tested, necessitating an experimental and a control group of subjects). Organ transplantation from a healthy to a sick person requires knowledge of the likely effects on both individuals and an attempt to measure the relative physiological gains and losses to both. The principle of "the sanctity of life" will be violated if the moral rules governing the attitude toward human bodies involuntarily threaten the integrity of those bodies as controlled by those to whom they belong.

As mentioned before, there is no end of dispute over rules of the kind sketched above. Some people, no doubt, would argue that I have not succeeded in accurately formulating the rules presently operating — at least those paid lip service to — in western culture; they may be right. There are also endless arguments about the way in which rules should be related to empirical data; about the degree to which rules should be understood as fixed absolutes, admitting of no exception; about the rights of individuals and groups to fix their own rules; about the value and relevance of the kind of typology I have offered here (is it really any help, for instance, to distinguish between "ethical principles" and "moral rules"?). Arguments of this kind are to

be expected and, in a time of rapidly changing medical technology, burgeoning life sciences, and shifting cultural values,
they are likely to be made all the more exasperating and bewil-
dering by a knowledge explosion the fruits of which are erratically, unevenly, and often obscurely disseminated and applied.

That much said by way of anticipating objections to my
analysis, let me nonetheless proceed to some further observations
and a possible way of effecting a synthesis. First, it can be seen
that each of the five rule systems I have abstractly distinguished
gives some measure of content to "the sanctity of life," but each
from a different angle. Thus "the sanctity of life" implies a spectrum of values ranging from the preservation of the species to
the inviolability of human bodies, from man in the aggregate
(present and future) to man as individual (present and future).
The discrete rule systems each serve an aspect of human life:
species-life; familial, lineage-life; body-life; person-life; and body
individuality-life. Each aspect of human life, therefore, has an
appropriate rule system designed to protect and foster that
aspect.

Secondly, though, it can be seen that the discrete rule systems overlap and together form a whole. One cannot talk for
long about rules designed to promote the survival of the human
species without eventually talking about their relationship to
rules governing familial lineage; decisions about the latter will influence the framing of the former, and vice versa. Nor can one
talk for long about species survival and lineage rules without
moving into a discussion of the integrity of personal individuality, with all that it implies about the right to procreate one's own
family, to make one's own choices and to act in ways affecting
the lives of others. These discussions in turn link up with rules
governing the right to bodily life in the first instance and to the
individual integrity of private bodies in the second. Even further,
however, a decision to grant everyone a guaranteed right to be
kept alive indefinitely by artificial means could, conceivably,
threaten the survival of the species, as could a decision to halt all
further medical experimentation on human subjects. An ill-con-
ceived rule in one area could inadvertently exert a harmful in-

fluence on the observance of rules in other areas; thus consistency and unity, as suggested before, are necessary for the totality of rules.

Perhaps this is only to state the obvious, but I think it worth stating since most recent attempts to cope with the new problems posed by advancing medical technology and life sciences are dealt with in almost total isolation from each other. Glanville Williams' otherwise fine book on *The Sanctity of Life and the Criminal Law* contains one detailed chapter after another on such subjects as abortion, euthanasia, contraception, and suicide. But each of these problems is presented as an independent concern [28]. He neither relates them to each other nor, for that matter, does he ever attempt to spell out the meaning of his usage of "the sanctity of life" and the way that usage ties his chapters together. Shils and Medawar, whom I have already cited, and even Paul Ramsey to a lesser extent, exhibit the same tendency. There is a large and growing literature on problems of life and death, but it is very rare, for instance, to find a discussion of when life begins creatively related to a discussion of when life ends. Yet clearly in that instance both problems turn on what is meant by "human life," and the illumination we gain in dealing with one of the problems will be useful when we deal with the other. Similarly, there is much to be said for trying to work for some consistent standards regarding the use of empirical data, standards which do not arbitrarily shift from one rule system to another [see 26]. Some of the older or now deceased ethicians — Catholic natural law thinkers, Maritain particularly; Barth, Brunner, and Bonhoeffer among Protestants — attempted to develop an encompassing theory to unite different rule systems. Yet most of their work was done before the advent of recent technological and medical developments, and, in any case, with the decline in emphasis among Catholic theologians on natural law theory [see 9], and among Protestants on systems of applied ethics, the trend is toward treating particular problems as *ad hoc* conundrums or to deal with the most abstract principles and ethical foundations only [19].

If my point is granted that the rule systems do inevitably overlap, and that indeed, it is helpful to seek out and utilize their connections, it should also be clear that some of the most difficult moral dilemmas are those which bring the different rules or rule systems in apparent conflict with each other. Rules granting individuals procreative rights can conflict with rules governing the welfare and survival of the species (as in overpopulated countries). Rules governing abortion can conflict with rules granting women the right not to procreate involuntarily. Rules controlling the (expensive) preservation of moribund individuals can conflict with the rights of families of those individuals to economic survival. Examples do not need to be multiplied; they are easily imaginable and very common.

One solution to such conflicts is to rank different rule systems (and their attendant rights and duties) in some kind of hierarchical order. Traditionally, I would suppose, the right to bodily life has taken precedence over other rights, though this precedence has admitted the exceptions which may be required when, as in wartime, other rights come to the fore. The reason for this precedence, as a general though not absolute ordering, has undoubtedly been the common sense perception that an essential condition for the exercise of human rights is the existence of human beings as the subjects of these rights; if one is not alive, all the rest is beside the point. But the ranking of rule systems and rights in a hierarchical order even in theory is complicated and in practice will obviously be conditioned by changing historical circumstances. Another solution would be to refuse any ranking of rule systems and to depend instead upon a testing of the conflicting rules together in the light of the principle of "the sanctity of life." But it is by no means evident that this would be very helpful; on the contrary, direct reliance upon the principle as such would not resolve conflicts. The principle only comes into play in the preliminary formation and final testing of rules and rule systems. The relationship between rules and systems will have to be worked out at the level of the rules themselves, or by recourse to a combination of other pertinent ethical principles — the principles of "least suffering," "lesser evil," and the like. If conflicting rules each serve the sanctity of life, then a choice which gives priority of one over the other could still serve and pass the final test of the principle; but knowing that much would be to know very little and thus require some other means of ordering the relationship of the rules.

SOME REGULATIVE OBSERVATIONS

Without pretending to offer anything approaching a complete solution to the ordering of rules, some regulative observations are in order, which may prove helpful. The first of these is that it is unlikely that a fixed ordering could be worked out which would be good for all times and in all circumstances. The setting of human life changes, influenced by a wide range of ecological, psychological, and economic considerations, to mention only a few. As suggested, the claim of the individual's "right to life" as the preeminent rule seems well-founded. Yet it is clearly conceivable that this right, and the attendant rules protecting it, could come into question if the survival of a whole people or nation were in danger from overpopulation, a scarcity of medical facilities, or in time of war. At such historical moments, a reordering of the rules could seem compellingly necessary; some hard decisions would be called for. Not only might the rules governing the individual's "right to life" come into difficult times, but also, consequently, all of the rule systems bearing on different aspects of the sanctity of life. A community or a nation could, naturally, decide to abide by some fixed, traditional ranking of the rule systems. It could decide that the right to individual life was so basic that, rather than permit abridgment, it would prefer a communal demise. It might well argue that a communal or national life which placed individual life in constant jeopardy would be a communal life not worth living. Yet it could as a community also come to a different conclusion: that communal survival was worth some restrictions on the individual's right to life. The abandonment of the elderly in earlier Eskimo culture, as well as the practice of infanticide in a variety of primitive societies, testifies to the extreme pressures which can be placed upon communal survival. To see such practices only as an instance of a primitive insensitivity to human life would be, I think, to show a lack of imagination about the kinds of desperate straits in which a community could find itself. It is surely not inconceivable that equally desperate situations could arise once again, even in our own day, and that communal decisions would have to be made offensive to our present ordering of rules.

A second observation is related to the first, and is even more important. Throughout this paper I have spoken of the relationship between the principle of "the sanctity of life" and the rules subsumed under it as a relationship of implication, i.e., "the sanctity of life" implies a variety of different rules governing the existence and integrity of human life. I want to argue that "implies" is the strongest concept that should be used to state the relationship: it means a relationship less binding than that of logical entailment. By "logical entailment" I mean a relationship between principle and rules which sees the particular rules as a strict deductive consequence of an affirmation of the principle. For instance, to say that an acceptance of "the sanctity of life" automatically requires, as part of its inherent *meaning*, a flat rule against the taking of individual human life, would be to see the relationship between principle and rule as one of logical entailment. On the contrary, I want to contend that the principle does not and should not function in this fashion, that it is sufficient to speak more loosely of specific rules being *implied* rather than *entailed* by the principle. Here I mean by "implied" a bias or a propensity toward certain kinds of rules, rules which would seem generally *reasonable* in light of the principle but not self-evident from a simple inspection of the principle itself. Thus it is eminently reasonable to see the principle implying a rule about the "right to life," but, once we are aware of the possibility of situations arising where this rule might have to be abridged in the interests of survival of the species, or survival of a whole people, we would realize that exceptions might have to be made to the rule. To make exceptions or, more precisely, to let other rules — e.g., those pertaining to species survival — take precedence could be, in some circumstances, to act reasonably. But if the relationship between principle and rule was one of entailment only, rigidly conceived, then the limits of reasonable moral choice would be preempted from the outset. In addition, once we realize that the different rules can at times conflict, we are forced to further realize that the principle, to be helpful, must leave us free to come to the most reasonable conclusion we can concerning the relative ordering of the rules. If the principle entailed only one ordering of the rules, or entailed only one possible choice in a moral dilemma, our freedom to act reasonably would be seriously restricted.

[The glaring weakness of Pope Paul's encyclical on birth control, *Humanae Vitae*, was his presumption, badly defended, that the protection of all human life entails an absolute prohibition against the use of contraceptives; no room was left for responsible choice.]

For all these reasons, the relationship between principle and rules should be kept flexible, sensitive to changing human contexts and shifting human needs (communal and individual). The principle best serves and judges us when it points us in a certain direction, inclines us to form certain kinds of rules, and instills a strong bias in favor of human life. As a test, it functions most fruitfully not when it logically binds us by a fixed set of logical implications, but when it forces us to look at the general trend of our rules and, on occasion, forces us to ask whether a given rule *really* serves the respect we want to accord human life. If the relationship between principle and rules was only one of strict logical implication, then nothing would require us to interrogate human experience; morality would then become solely a matter of explicating the given linguistic meaning of principle and rules to see whether the relationship between these meanings was one of logical entailment. As a procedure for coming to moral decisions that would seem to me inadmissible.

There is an even more important aspect of this last problem, particularly as it bears on religious explanations of the source and meaning of "the sanctity of life." Peter Berger has wisely pointed out that "Whatever the 'ultimate' merits of religious explanations of the universe at large, their empirical tendency has been to falsify man's consciousness of that part of the universe shaped by his own activity, namely, the socio-cultural world" [5:90]. One way in which a religious explanation of "the sanctity of life" can lead to a falsification of consciousness is when it is taken to suggest that man's moral rules are not of his own making, but have, somehow, been imposed upon him by God. The weakness in a narrow natural law philosophy is less its much-condemned legalism than its tendency to act as if God has *disclosed* to man a set of inflexible moral rules which man has only to discern and obey. A Christian biblical fundamentalism shows the same tendencies, substituting the supposed direct deliverances of revelation for the propositions of natural law theory. The result in either case is falsification of consciousness: laws and rules believed by men of an earlier era to have been reasonable rules of conduct are transmuted by later generations into set, transcendent codes. As it happens, the fact that in practice rigid codes very often admit of multitudinous exceptions and extenuating circumstances testifies to the meliorating impact of experience and conflict among basic values. (1) "Thou shalt not kill" — unless (2) one kills in a legitimate war, in self-defense, in imposing lawful capital punishment, and so on. The first is the rigid rule, the second is the accepted understanding of that rule. The falsification of consciousness arises when, despite the conceded exceptions, the rules are still treated as "God-given," either through reason or revelation. That even rigid codes have been forced to admit exceptions and complexities should actually make clear that all moral rules are human artifacts. The fiction of divinely imposed rules does justice neither to the moral rules nor to God. Justice is not done to the rules because their character as guides to and exemplars of higher ethical principles rather than rigid entailments of these principles is obscured. Justice is not done to God because it is presupposed that God's moral relationship to man is essentially that of law-giver, a less than rich relationship.

The way to avoid such a falsification of consciousness is by man's taking full responsibility for his own fate and that of others. The principle of "the sanctity of life," even if given a religious grounding, is best protected by the recognition that it is human beings who must form, implement, and set the conditions of those rules designed to protect and foster that sanctity. There are three reasons why this recognition is necessary.

First, as suggested in the discussion of the five rule systems, it is evident that man must define the terms of the rules, examine the data, and then make use of the data. The result of this complicated process will, inexorably, make the utilized rules *human* rules; it would be inappropriate to call them anything else after so many human judgments have been made in the process of interpreting and using them. To say, for instance, that God forbids the taking of "innocent" life, while conceding — as I think we must — that it is left up to man to define what an "innocent" life is, is to fail to see that the only possible *meaning* this rule could have is the meaning human beings *choose* to give it.

Second, it is an utter abdication of human responsibility to passively place on God's shoulders the care and protection of human life. Human experience together with a contemplation of human freedom and divine providence show that God does not directly enter into the processes of nature and human life, at least not in the sense of immediately intervening in the biological processes of life and death. With rare exceptions, Christian theology has always granted human beings the right to take those steps — scientific, moral, and technological — which they believe necessary for their safety, progress, and dignity. That it has done so is a tacit recognition that it is man who is responsible for man. I am only proposing that we carry the implication of this perception to its logical conclusion: man is responsible for everything to do with man, including control over life and death. This is the last step that much Christian theology has been slow to take, but it is now imperative. Contraception, abortion, euthanasia, medical experimentation, and the prolongation of human life are all problems which fall *totally* within the sphere of human rules and human judgments. To place the solution of these problems "in the hands of God" is to misjudge God's role and to misuse human reason and freedom.

It is often said that man can't "play God" with human life, that certain natural processes must be left entirely to God's providence. The trouble with that kind of moral reasoning is that it fails to see that God himself does not "play God" as that phrase is usually understood; that is, God does not directly and miraculously intervene in natural processes. He does not "bring" human beings into life or "make" them die, just as he doesn't "make" them sick or "cure" them of illness. The theology behind the excuse that man can't "play God" is a defective theology. Dr. Alan F. Guttmacher has an effective complaint: "When it comes to many of the social problems of medicine . . . sterilization, therapeutic abortion, donor artificial insemination, and withholding resuscitative techniques to seriously malformed infants in the delivery room — doctors retreat behind the cliché that they 'won't play God.' This type of intellectual cowardice, this mental retreat is irrational . . . through the nature of his work a doctor is constantly intruding himself into the work of the Deity. Does he wait for God to show his decision by making some outward manifestation before he undertakes a Caesarean section, orders a transfusion, or performs a risk-fraught open-heart operation" [15:458]? Martin J. Buss' proposal that "it is best to identify God's purposes with man's good as such, rather than with any specific process," is a wise one, for it helps make clear that man is responsible for himself and the world and, at the same time, it is consonant with more recent Catholic natural law thinking and Protestant responsibility ethics [7:250 ff].

My third reason for the recognition of human responsibilities relates to the first two. Perhaps the most vexing problem of medical ethics and the human uses of technology is what can be called "line-drawing." At what point in gestation are we to say that human life "begins" and thus (if we believe that to be the critical question), draw a line against abortion? At what point are we to say that "death" has occurred and thus feel free to transplant an organ or cease artificial organ support or resuscitation? Where do we draw the line in exposing subjects of medical experiments to mental or physical dangers? Even if we have very explicit formal rules, questions of this type are difficult to answer; the rules themselves do not answer them. They are a matter of human judgment. More than that, the need to draw lines, to set a limit to moral behavior, is a call to establish a moral policy. If we want to know when life "begins" or "ends," biological and other scientific knowledge will provide us with some clues — empirical data on which to base a judgment. But the value of this knowledge, its *meaning* for human use by human beings, will be a function of the human goals we want to achieve. Lines, in a word, do not draw themselves and scientific data will not of themselves draw lines for us. Decisions must be made about how we want to use the data, and these decisions will reflect our moral policy.

A moral policy decision to extend protection of individual human life to the utmost conceivable limit would, for instance, suggest drawing a line on the beginning of human life very early in the conception process and very late in the dying process. Another moral policy decision, however, might be one which sought to strike a balance between individual rights and the needs of a community to survive. In that case, the beginning of human life might be designated as taking place relatively late in gestation (making abortion permissible) and death as occurring relatively early in the dying process (making an early cessation of artificial support permissible). Each of these policy decisions, which could have different social consequences, presupposes that the scientific data as such are ambiguous enough to provide some margin of flexibility. The data on the gestational process are of little use to us unless we have a prior definition of "human life," just as data on the dying process require being set in the context of a prior definition of what we choose to call "human death." These definitions will also be part of moral policy decisions; they will influence our interpretation of the data, which, taken alone, would not necessarily suggest any particular policy. In saying this, I would still want to stress a point made earlier: just as our rules should be consistent with each other, our standards concerning the use of data should be consistent from one rule system to another. A method of using data to solve the abortion problem which was very different from the method used to solve the problem of sustaining moribund life ought to arouse our suspicion. It could suggest that one or the other of the methods, or perhaps both, was arbitrary. A consistent method of using data from one rule system to another provides some degree of protection against capriciousness, as well as a goad to disinterested interpretation of data.

SOME UNSOLVED PROBLEMS

In sketching the three reasons why I believe it necessary, indeed unavoidable, for human beings to take total responsibility for human life and death, I do not want to leave the impression that my approach solves all problems — far from it. One which it does not solve is that of the extent to which our humanly devised rules should be established as absolute moral rules. By and large, for the sake of achieving a moral consensus, our rules should be as clear as possible. This is particularly important when one person puts his body or life in the hands of another — clarity and commonly binding consensus help provide the basis for trust and security.. Our rules should also be capable of change if circumstances or changing moral evaluations point toward the need for change. At the same time, I think it imperative to avoid any theory of rules which would preclude human beings from establishing absolute, unbreakable rules, at least absolute for a time and under certain specified social conditions.

"Absolute taboos, with their underlying mystique about life," Joseph Fletcher has written, "make a farce of human freedom. All such taboos cut the ground out from under morality because nothing we do lies in the moral order if it is not humanly chosen" [11:63]. One can see what Professor Fletcher is driving at here, but some qualifications are in order. All "taboos," for one thing, need not spring from a "mystique about life." They could be the result of very rational decisions. For example, a community with a history of medical abuse and malpractice could decide that the dangers of leaving decisions about the prolongation of moribund life in the hands of individual doctors and families had become so great as to dictate an absolute rule requiring doctors to take every possible step to prolong life, however extraordinary. This kind of rule could of course be very cumbersome to observe in some cases, but a community might decide that, for the value of affording patients a greater sense of security when in the hands of doctors, it would be a desirable rule. A "taboo" against genocide, to choose another example, would not appear irrational. Absolute pacifism, while it has not commended itself to most men, is not an insane position. It is simply the conviction that an absolute rule against war — a "taboo," if you will — would be a wise rule, even in cases of legitimate self-defense. The reasoning behind this position is that human experience shows (or in the eyes of the pacifists shows) that all wars, even just wars, have bad consequences; hence, an absolute refusal to engage in war is required. For another thing, to take Prof. Fletcher's point, if his standard is "human choice," I see no reason why a "human choice" in favor of "absolute taboos" in some circumstances should be ruled out a priori. The important consideration, I should think, would be its character as a "human choice," i.e., reasonable, sensitive, imaginative. A "taboo" which displayed this character could be a very wise one (even if open to debate).

Another problem which my approach does not solve is that of telling us exactly how we should go about establishing those moral policies which will shape our rule systems and influence our use of data. To do that would require a further paper. But I think I have said enough to indicate the general lines of an approach. Our policy decisions, and the consequent moral rules developed together with further procedural rules for ordering and relating the moral rules, must take account of the "whole man." By that I mean man from the beginning to the end of his life, as an individual and as a member of a species and a community, as the subject of bodily and intellectual rights. This is only to say that all our rules must be congruent with each other, and our overall policy coherent and orderly. The final measure of our moral policy and its attendant rules will be the principle of "the sanctity of life." There is no final test of this principle. In affirming it, we go as far as we can in trying to articulate an ultimate ethical norm against which all other norms must be measured. Beyond a commitment to this principle there is only what Professor Aiken has called the "post-ethical" level of moral discourse. That is the level at which we move out of ethics altogether to choose a worldview [1:83 ff]. Suppose someone asks "Why ought I to respect the sanctity of life, or even suppose there is such a principle?" It is unlikely we could even begin to give him a convincing answer if he did not share with us some common assumptions or commitments about the nature of everything which exists. There comes a point in moral discourse and human reasoning beyond which we cannot go without an infinite regress or without circling back to where we began. At that point, Aiken correctly notes, "Decision is king" [1:87].

The direction of my own decision and, I trust, of most human beings, is to affirm the value of the principle of "the sanctity of life." James Gustafson, though operating from within a Christian framework, has written what I would hope to be acceptable outside of that framework: "Life is to be preserved, the weak and the helpless are to be cared for especially, the moral requisites of trust, hope, love, freedom, justice, and others are to be met so that human life can be meaningful. This bias gives a direction . . ." [14].

REFERENCES

1. Aiken, Henry D: Levels of Moral Discourse, in *Reason and Conduct* (Alfred A Knopf, New York, New York) 1962.
2. Barker, S F: *Induction and Hypothesis* (Cornell University Press, Ithaca, New York) 1957.
3. Barth, Karl: *Church Dogmatics*, vol III/4, par 55, p 355 (T and T Clark, Edinburgh, Scotland) 1961, cited in Paul Ramsey: The Morality of Abortion, in Daniel H Labby, ed: *Life or Death: Ethics and Options* (University of Washington Press, Seattle, Washington) 1968, p 75.
4. Beecher, Henry K: Medical Research and the Individual, in

Daniel H Labby, ed: *Life or Death: Ethics and Options* (University of Washington Press, Seattle, Washington) 1968, a sensitive confrontation of a number of the problems arising in sections (d) and (e).

5. Berger, Peter L: *The Sacred Canopy* (Doubleday & Co, Inc, Garden City, New York) 1967.
6. Bonhoeffer, Dietrich, *Ethics*, Neville Horton Smith, translator (SCM Press, London, England) 1955.
7. Buss, Martin J: The Beginning of Life as an Ethical Problem, *The Journal of Religion*, July 1967.
8. Cairns, David: *God Up There?* (Westminster Press, Philadelphia, Pennsylvania) 1967.
9. Curran, Charles E: Absolute Norms and Medical Ethics, in Charles E Curran, ed: *Absolutes in Moral Theology* (Corpus Books, Washington, D.C.) 1968.
10. Death. For some medical discussions see Halley, M Martin, and Harvey, William J: Medical vs Legal Definition of Death, *Journal of the American Medical Association*, vol 204, May 6, 1968, pp 423–425; Hamlin, Hannibal: Life or Death by EEG, *Journal of the American Medical Association*, vol 190, Oct 12, 1964, pp 112–114; Negovsky, V A: Some Physiopathic Regularities in the Process of Dying and Resuscitation, *Circulation*, vol XXIII, March, 1961, pp 452–457; *Journal of the American Medical Association*, vol 204, May 6, 1968, p 539, editorial. For some theological treatments see *Decisions About Life and Death* (Church Assembly Board for Social Responsibility, London, England) 1965; Pius XII: allocution to a congress of anesthetists, Nov 24, 1957, in *Acta Apostolicae Sedis*, vol XLIX, 1957, pp 1027–1033; Nolan, Kieran: The Problem of Care for the Dying, in Charles E Curran, ed: *Absolutes in Moral Theology* (Corpus Books, Washington, D.C.) 1968, pp 249–260.
11. Fletcher, Joseph: The Right to Die, *Atlantic Monthly*, Apr 1968.
12. Fuchs, Josef, SJ: *Natural Law*, Helmut Reckter, SJ, and John A Dowling, translators (Sheed & Ward, New York, New York) 1965.

13. Genetics. For two good surveys and discussions see Osborn, Frederick: *The Future of Human Heredity* (Weybright and Talley, New York, New York) 1968; Hirschhorn, Kurt: Genetics: Re-Doing Man, *Commonweal*, May 17, 1968, pp 257–261. The leading exponent of positive eugenics is Muller, H J: Genetic Progress by Voluntarily Controlled Germinal Choice, in G Wolstenholne, ed: *Man and His Future* (Little, Brown & Co, Boston, Massachusetts) 1967, pp 247–262. A position favoring negative eugenics is taken by Medawar, P B: Genetic Options: An Examination of Current Fallacies, in Daniel H Labby, ed: *Life or Death: Ethics and Options* (University of Washington Press, Seattle, Washington) 1968. Several positions are examined in Manier, Edward: Genetics and the Future of Man: Scientific and Ethical Possibilities, *Proceedings of the American Catholic Philosophical Association*, 1968, forthcoming.

14. Gustafson, James F: A Christian Approach to the Ethics of Abortion, unpublished paper delivered at Harvard Divinity School / Kennedy Foundation Symposium on Abortion, Washington, D.C., Aug 1967.

15. Guttmacher, Alan F: The United States Medical Profession and Family Planning, in Bernard Berelson, ed: *Family Planning and Population Programs* (University of Chicago Press, Chicago, Illinois) 1966.

16. Häring, Bernard: *The Law of Christ*, vol III (Newman Press, Westminster, Maryland) 1965.

17. Hick, John: *Evil and the Love of God* (Harper and Row, New York, New York) 1966, the best recent book on the problem of evil.

18. Kelly, Gerald: *Medico-Moral Problems* (Clonmore and Reynolds, Dublin, Ireland) 1955.

19. Lehmann, Paul: *Ethics in a Christian Context* (Harper and Row, New York, New York) 1963, an outstanding book dealing with ethical problems.

20. Medawar, P B: Genetic Options: An Examination of Current Fallacies, in Daniel H Labby, ed: *Life or Death: Ethics*

and Options (University of Washington Press, Seattle, Washington) 1968.

21. Ramsey, Paul: The Morality of Abortion, in Daniel H Labby, ed: *Life or Death: Ethics and Options* (University of Washington Press, Seattle, Washington) 1968.

22. St John-Stevas, Norman: Law and the Moral Consensus, in Daniel H Labby, ed: *Life or Death: Ethics and Options* (University of Washington Press, Seattle, Washington) 1968.

23. St John-Stevas, Norman: *The Right to Life* (Holt, Rinehart and Winston, New York, New York) 1964.

24. Schöllgen, Werner: *Moral Problems Today*, Edward Quinn, translator (Herder and Herder, New York, New York) 1963.

25. Shils, Edward: The Sanctity of Life, in Daniel H Labby, ed: *Life or Death: Ethics and Options* (University of Washington Press, Seattle, Washington) 1968.

26. Stackhouse, Max L: Technical Data and Ethical Norms, *Journal for the Scientific Study of Religion*, vol V, Spring 1966, pp 191–203.

27. Thielicke, Helmut: *The Ethics of Sex*, John W Doberstein, translator (Harper and Row, New York, New York) 1964.

28. Williams, Glanville: *The Sanctity of Life and the Criminal Law* (Faber and Faber, London, England) 1958

COMMENTARY

by *Julian R. Pleasants*

DANIEL CALLAHAN has tackled head-on the crucial problem of our time, and especially of our country. The particular ethical problems raised by recent medical research are dramatic and headline catching, but they are not really new, nor are they major threats to the sanctity of life. The major threats are still war, malnutrition, disease, abortion, inequitable trade balances, maldistribution of resources, and the like. What scientific and medical discoveries have done is to bring into sharp focus, and to bring home to our affluent society, the kinds of manipulation of human life that we have already been doing, indirectly and often unconsciously. Mr. Callahan has done an especially valuable job of showing that it will not do to answer the apparently new medical problems on an *ad hoc* basis or on the basis of particular religious traditions or by means of political deals and pressures. I would like to second this by indicating how any clarification of our attitude toward the sanctity of life will be of critical importance, not only for solving the more exotic problems of medical experimentation, but for meeting the real gut issues of our world. American and Soviet societies have assumed almost without question that we can increase indefinitely the quality of our own lives by means of policies which threaten the very survival of other people's lives, and which may ultimately threaten our own. From the biologist's point of view, man appears to be rushing down one of evolution's blind alleys.

Not man only, but many animal species as well owe their survival to the way they respect the lives of their fellow species members. Very often this respect shows itself in a strange (to us) mixture of aggressive attack with inhibitions which stop the attack short of injury or death. Through this mixture the species obtains the survival value of aggressive instincts: spacing of animals, stimulation of physical and mental development, selection of strong partners for mating, and development of cooperative bonds and hierarchical relationships which make possible group life and group defense against all hazards. Yet the animal species obtains these without decimating its numbers. In very few species in nature is the weaker animal killed; instead, the one which fails in a test of strength shows a sign of surrender which is accepted as such by the stronger party. It is a ritual conflict. Only in captivity, where the loser cannot go away, will a battle of two animals go on to the death of the loser. A rat clan will kill an intruder from another clan without giving him a chance to retreat to his own territory, but this is an exceptional species.

Only among men is it common for one individual to kill another. And it is unique to man for one group deliberately to decimate or destroy another group. According to one psychological theory it is not that man has more aggressive drives than other species, but that his aggressive actions have been made vastly more lethal by the invention of weapons. Inhibitions against killing a fellow species member seem inoperative or less operative in man than in other animal species, either because their genetic base has disappeared or because the instinctive inhibitions don't have a chance to come into play as they might in weaponless combat. Within the group with which a man identifies — his family, village, and nation — he does respect the lives of his fellow men. Bonds have been formed that keep him from attacking his own group. If he were not basically more cooperative than hostile, man could not survive; he is too dependent on culture for his survival. Even in the group with which he has bonds, however, a man's inhibitions are probably less effective when he has a weapon in his hand (an important point in the gun control controversy). Between groups of men, however, human hostility seems to be under few inhibitions, quite unlike animal species. Even animals which reserve all their aggression for the "other" group still have inhibitions against killing the others. War is a peculiarly human pastime.

In fact, as human aggressive actions have become more lethal, and inhibitions against killing less effective, it has become more and more the case that the only good defense is a good offense. There has therefore been strong selection pressure (an evolutionist's term for increased chance of survival and reproduction) for groups which were more warlike, whether for genetic or cultural reasons. This may mean that man has entered one of evolution's blind alleys, in which selection pressure can push him in only one direction, toward his own extermination. This has happened to other species in which the major selection pressure on the species was for some characteristic used for battle within the species. The Irish elk became extinct when its antlers, used only for the males' testing of each other, became increasingly heavy and awkward. Some other species seem to be traveling similar blind alleys right now. The human species, however, had become so numerous and widespread that it hardly seemed possible that it could eliminate itself through an unbalanced pressure for aggression. The nuclear age has suddenly made that possibility of self-extermination seem a real one. Unless mankind can reach some consensus about the sanctity of human life, not only within groups of humans, but between groups — unless it can divert or ritualize its aggressive tendencies into something non-lethal — it may commit the ultimate biological sin for any species, self-extermination. Even without going that far, man has it in his power to destroy a vast amount of human life and human potential, both genetic and cultural.

In this as in other cases, scientific and medical research have not really created new problems; they have simply magnified the old ones to such proportions that we can no longer ignore them. We have had genetic engineering, for example, as long as we have had marriage systems (polygamy, monogamy, inbreeding, outbreeding, segregation), as long as we've sent young men out to die before they could reproduce, as long as couples have been paired up for any reasons other than pure chance, and as long as couples have decided how many children they will contribute to the next generation. But modern science makes the further possibilities seem awesome. My own research in developing liquid diets for infant germ-free animals could prepare the way for raising a fetus in an artificial medium, perhaps from conception. In other lines of biological research, a whole new organism has been grown from a single *body* cell (not a reproductive cell) of another organism. The possibility looms of growing 10,000 individuals, genetically identical, from the body cells of one individual, as well as modifying genes by various treatments before starting development in the artificial medium. *Brave New World* is closer than we think, and the responsibility should very properly awe us. But we have already chosen genetic engineering in principle.

It is not transplants and artificial kidneys which created the problem of deciding who should live and who should die. As long as we have had effective medical treatments for dangerous diseases, but not enough treatment to go around, we have been deciding who should live and who should die — but we have been leaving it up to money to decide, that of the nation or of the individual. It didn't take the development of hallucinogens to put personality control in our grasp. Obviously we have been changing personalities by segregation and ghettos for some time. But also, as long as Americans have fed their high protein grains to meat animals instead of shipping them to tropical countries, we have condemned millions of children to irreversible physical and mental retardation and to permanent lethargy. But we share this responsibility with their parents and their parents' spiritual leaders, Catholic, Hindu, and Communist, when these promote a rate of population growth which would soon eat up the carrying capacity of America's extra acres.

What scientific advancement has suddenly brought home to white America is the possibility of doing things to each other, *within* our group, that we have been doing indirectly and even unconsciously to those outside our group, deciding who shall live and who shall die and who shall half-live, manipulating people by the way we manipulate the tremendous resources of land, energy, and talent which we have managed to keep at our disposal. We stand at a kind of moral crossroads. Having realized what we *can* do to our own group and what we *have been* doing to other groups, we may decide to keep two different standards of respect for life; we may decide to extend to insiders our present attitude toward outsiders, or we may decide to extend to outsiders our present attitude toward insiders.

The demand for an extreme liberalization of abortion rules seems to me an example of one road: extension to insiders of an attitude toward life developed for outsiders. The bombardier about to loose his bombs on a Vietnamese village may be able to see figures scurrying about below, but they are so tiny and shapeless that he cannot *see* them as human beings, though he may have indirect reasons to think so. He would rather not kill them, but they could be a threat to a way of life; they are or could be troublemakers. Besides, their lives seem so primitive and unimportant. It takes only the touch of a button to eliminate them and he won't even see it happen. What chance is there for instinctive inhibitions to operate either in aerial warfare or in abortion? The hostility hitherto reserved for our enemies can now be visited on our own children, who seem as much a threat to the quality of our lives as does the outside agitator who demands a share of what we have.

And, *de facto*, it is true. The measure of our respect for the sanctity of life is what we are willing to take from the quality of our lives in order that others may live. Yet the specter of overpopulation has given us very ambivalent feelings about making sacrifices so that others may live. I know very well that the cost of my second car would buy someone a lifesaving operation, and that the cost of my recreations would save at least one and perhaps many Latin American infants from starvation. Yet I don't know how to balance the moral books on such a choice. The kind of discussion which Mr. Callahan pursues is essential if the moral sense of America is to be awakened. Does maintaining and increasing the American standard of living take precedence over the lives and aspirations of other groups? In an interdependent world, the rights of one are hollow shams if they entail no responsibility to the rights of others. Yet how far does that responsibility go; how much does it demand of me? These are some of the psychological hurdles that a consensus on the sanctity of life must be able to surmount.

Yet if man is to surmount those hurdles and even take the road of giving outsiders' lives the same respect he gives to insiders' lives, if he is to escape the blind alley of megaweapon warfare down which natural selection seems to be propelling him, what psychological forces does he have going for him? Can the same reasoning power which forged such weapons produce a consensus to save us from them and from the other awesome opportunities for human manipulation and destruction which may become available? Reason can redirect, but can it provide the motivational energy to carry man in the new direction? How can man extend the bonds he has within his own groups to include outside groups? In fact, if you take away the hostility of outside groups, can he even maintain the bonds he has formed within his own group? It will take a profound understanding of human psychology to answer these questions effectively. Many efforts to forge such bonds are already being made and others can be suggested, but I would like to concentrate on one as especially relevant to the context of this discussion.

It has become unfashionable to credit Christianity with any important role in human evolution. And I am as unable as Mr. Callahan to find any evidence of a Divine providence constantly meddling in human affairs or in the natural world. I can fully agree with him that man's role in the world is to "play God"; otherwise the role will not be played. Yet the coming of Jesus Christ into human history seems to me to have given human evolution a new direction — that of according *all* men the respect reserved hitherto for one's own group. The fact that so many men of the West recognize this as the ideal, even while their policies work against it, represents to me an achievement, however incomplete, of this new direction in human evolution, a new direction which can save man from the blind forces of natural selection.

Other forces can work in that new direction as well, including our fear of nuclear war, of massive malnutrition, and of ideological tyranny. New communications media help. All available forces must be used. At the moment it is not at all clear that Christian leadership retains enough force in human affairs to act as a strong selection pressure. Certainly papal influence (as of August, 1968) is at a new low, but this may create the opportunity for a new kind of Catholic leadership to emerge. In the civil rights movement, in its concern over Vietnam, Christian leadership has shown a new capacity for redirecting itself and others towards its own ideal of universal brotherhood. I do not for a moment disagree with Mr. Callahan's thesis that we must have a non-religious basis for consensus about the sanctity of human life. Reason can see the indivisibility of human welfare, and can recognize that no one is safe unless everyone is safe, even while we are struggling with the unspoken feeling that in an overpopulated world individual lives are not so terribly important. The basic human motives that enable a man to love and sacrifice for his own group can be extended, if we can find out how. But I see a crucial role for Christian love in helping to induce that extension, motivating pyschological explorations and rational discussions like that of Mr. Callahan. I see Christianity doing this as part of a generally secular movement, yet without jettisoning the unique motivational force it derives from the good news of a loving God, and its correlative, the promise of personal resurrection. The Christian gospel of universal brotherhood could be the indispensable, though not the sole, corrective for the tragic flaw in man's biological constitution.

REFERENCE

1. Lorenz, Konrad: *On Aggression* (Harcourt, Brace & World, New York, New York) 1966.

COMMENTARY
by James M. Gustafson

CALLAHAN HAS SEVERAL intentions in his article that are worth noting. First, he is obviously seeking to define both a normative principle and some procedures of ethical thinking which avoid the wastelands of absolute relativism on the one hand, and the narrow rigors of legalism on the other. Second, he is responding to current literature which deals with the question of the sanctity of life in an appreciative and yet critical way. Third, he wishes to be of some practical assistance to those who have the power and responsibility to make judgments and to act in circumstances in which the moral questions of life's value become concrete. Like any writing with these intentions, this one evokes responses both to the methods involved and to the normative ethics espoused. I shall not make a point by point detailed analysis of his arguments, but rather indicate some of the issues which remain outstanding when he has finished. Some of them are developed directly from his article; some constitute "further observations."

Callahan involves himself in one vast issue which does not get the detailed treatment it merits: the ultimate justification for the normative principles which embody the positive moral value of the sanctity of life. He deals with Edward Shils' essay in *Life or Death: Ethics and Options* in a sympathetic way, for Callahan seeks to find a foundation for general acceptance of the sanctity of life that is not tied to a particular religious history or to traditional conceptions of natural law but to some grounding in experience. Shils is interesting on this issue, for he appears to believe that life has been valued in western culture because of the moral and historical influences of the western religions. Yet the religions themselves are no longer acceptable. Thus, in my reading, he somewhat plaintively seeks to find out what functions these religions have had which made them value life. If this can be determined, we might find what underlies them which is of universal human acceptance. It appears to be a kind of primitive natural response.

The question in ethical theory which emerges is this: do the foundations in belief, whether religiously or rationally justified, which support a moral value of sanctity of life in any way affect the judgments made about it in particular cases? Or are these merely the kinds of justifying frameworks that people formulate in order to give an ultimate reason for what seems to be a social necessity or a commonly accepted human moral value? It is clear that one does not have to have a Jewish or Christian theology in order to value human life. But does a Jewish or Christian theology which supports the moral principles which protect life in any way set limits, safeguards, or restrictions to what men are permitted to do with other human lives? Historically, religious systems have not had a single effect in this regard. Catholic resistance to changes in the moral and legal rules on a matter like abortion seems to be an exception, but the value of life's sanctity has not been upheld with equal rigor by Catholics in other areas of human moral life such as capital punishment, war, and the like. But to indicate the ambiguity of historical evidence does not in itself answer the more normative question: Are there limits to man's tampering with human life which have a more direct relationship to religious beliefs? If there are, this would not mean that there are no principles upon which religious men could agree with others as to limits established regarding most potential circumstances. It would, however, force more systematically than Callahan does in this essay the question of the practical consequences of the particular ultimate foundations one might establish for the morality of the care of human life.

A second issue emerges from Callahan's essay. It regards simply words at one level, but their significance is greater than their simplicity. Is it best to speak of the "sanctity" of life? Callahan suggests some other terms, for example, "dignity," "ultimate value," "worth," "significance," and "importance." Notably, when he is expounding his system of rules, another term crops up, namely "rights." What difference might it make to a discussion like Callahan's if the primary language was the "right to life" rather than the "sanctity of life"? I believe it could make a considerable difference, because in function "sanctity" often translates out as "value" rather than as "right." Insofar as it does, not only in this essay but in the writings of others (including myself), a predisposition has been established which proceeds to calculate various values and to make a judgment which will be based largely on the potential consequences of alternative courses of action. We begin to set the problem in terms of competing and conflicting moral values, usually in terms of some general notion of whether there will be an increment in human well-being communally. Then we begin to assess what positive values can be sacrificed for others. If, however, we speak primarily of the "right to life," there is a different set of accents to the discussion. Callahan's five points that rules must attend to are interesting in this regard. Four of the five have their delineation in terms of the protection of rights, e.g., "neither the state nor individuals have the right to (unjustly) deprive human beings of their lives," as a development of his (c), the integrity of bodily life. The parenthetical "unjustly" is the nub of the matter, of course. It raises the large question of how justice is to be understood, whether in terms of certain consequences which might enhance general well-being, or in its own "rights" terms.

The matter has practical consequences when the ethics of abortion are discussed. If one speaks of the fetus's "right to life," it is more difficult to justify an abortion than if one speaks of the value of the life of the fetus in relation to a whole host of other values which might be jeopardized to some degree if the fetus is permitted to live. Fetuses have no significant utility value; mothers have a great deal of utility value. Unless one speaks of the intrinsic value of the fetus being equal to the intrinsic value of the mother, each having fundamentally an inalienable right to bodily existence, it becomes easier to find the value considerations which might make the death of the fetus morally viable. It is the weight of considerations which press more heavily when one speaks of the *right* to live that those who readily translate "sanctity" out as "value" sometimes avoid. It is more difficult to defend an "overriding right" than it is to defend the mathematics that often goes into the calculation of values in relation to each other. One might even end up with deontological ethics.

A third issue which Callahan's article deals with at great length is the relation between general ethical principles and particular moral rules. Here he shows more methodological sophistication than Protestant writers have generally had, though he does not proceed in the same fashion as his fellow Catholics have in the past. He takes his cues from Henry David Aiken's discussion of the levels of moral discourse, though he revises it for his purposes. Callahan has a double relationship between particular moral rules and general ethical principles: "the rules give content, on a lower level, to the principles; the principle, on a higher level, is used to judge the rules." Of course, he fills this statement out and does much more, including making the effort to have rules which are consistent with one another.

The literature on this topic, of course, is very extensive. Among American moral philosophers one thinks of John Rawls,

Marcus Singer, Richard Brandt, Kurt Baier, and others; among Protestant theologians, Paul Ramsey. Callahan's discussion has more practical bite to it than some of the philosophical writings, precisely because he is engaged in an exercise of the practical reason to indicate some possible ways to come to agreement on a particular issue.

It is not a negative judgment against his treatment to indicate that the reflections might have had more connections with a number of moral philosophers if he had dealt with the question of "universalizability" directly and head-on. There is debate as to whether "generalizability" is not a preferable term, but whichever term one uses, the question raises useful points when pursuing the principles and rules issues. Marcus Singer, for example, writes about the generalization issue in two ways. He calls the generalization "argument" the effects of the simple question, "What would happen if everyone did that? . . . If the consequences of everyone's acting in a certain way would be undesirable, then it would be wrong for anyone to act in that way." The generalization "principle," Singer states as follows, "What is right for one person must be right for any similar person in similar circumstances" [2:162–163; see 1]. Singer goes on to show how the generalization argument "serves to generate and establish" moral rules and in part determines "the range of their application," and also serves to mediate between rules when they conflict. One could get into questions of terminology very readily, but that would be beside the point here. The point is to suggest that 1) what Callahan calls a "principle" is perhaps more laden with normative ethical content than what some others would want a principle to be, and that 2) it would have been interesting to see Callahan explore his normative principle in the light of the generalizability question.

Matters of the logical connections between principles and rules are much explored these days. I shall only call attention to Callahan's awareness of the issues as being a salutary one, for much writing which has even as limited a practical intention as his does blithely ignores the kinds of questions which moral philosophers are raising, questions which are of practical as well as theoretical significance. I would also call attention to the way in which Callahan is aware of the issues involved in using technical scientific data in making moral judgments. This, too, is an area of more intricate discussion than can be explored at this point: it involves the fact-value question, the understanding of the relation of circumstances to moral judgments and actions and a wide range of other issues.

Finally, by way of "further observations," I would note a more subjective issue, namely to what extent will arguments about the sanctity of life be persuasive when the fundamental disposition or attitude of respect for, or reverence for, life is not secure. The latter words are chosen with care; I do not wish to indicate that I believe there is a fundamental decline in the reverence or respect for life, nor do I wish to indicate that the situation is satisfactory from a moral point of view. One can easily observe, as others have done, contradictory tendencies within the societies of the world. In American life there is growing repugnance in some circles at the thought of capital punishment and chemical warfare and killing. At the same time other tendencies are present; we are as callous now about automobile traffic deaths as persons in the past were about deaths due to diseases which have been largely conquered, and we have the persistent problem of violence. No doubt there are many pacifists and anti-capital punishment people who are in favor of the liberalization of abortion laws beyond the recommendations of the Model Penal Code. Invasions of privacy become subtle and technically brilliant. Ours is not a society in which one can depend upon reverence for life being subjectively present in the whole population.

This only points to the deeper spiritual problem. Is the confusion about the reverence for life in any way related to man's capacity to determine his own destiny, to his acceptance of moral responsibility for his own acts, to his loss of a sense of the transcendent? Is a loss of the sense of the reverence for life an inevitable accompaniment of growing secularization? What are the conditions which would make for a profounder subjective respect for life? When our ethical thinking becomes so objectified that we attend only to the rational bases for making moral judgments, and forget that judgments are also conditioned by fundamental attitudes and dispositions toward other human beings, we may have won some points, but we have not yet won the game.

REFERENCES

1. Singer, Marcus: *Generalization in Ethics* (Alfred A Knopf, Inc, New York, New York) 1961.
2. Singer, Marcus: Moral Rules and Principles, in A. I. Melden, ed: *Essays in Moral Philosophy* (University of Washington Press, Seattle, Washington) 1958.

COMMENTARY

by Henry K. Beecher

I AM INDEBTED to Mr. Callahan for giving me a much clearer understanding of just what the concept "the sanctity of life" can mean. A few years ago I took part in a symposium at Reed College on this theme. It seemed then that this phrase was no more than an expression of a goal toward which we can and must strive, but a goal without any true meaning in terms of likely consequences of the striving. I have a different view now.

The principle of the sanctity of life subsumes certain rules by implication. It implies "a bias or propensity toward certain kinds of rules. . . ." There is the "right to life"; there is the "right to be let alone" in Judge Cooley's memorable phrase [4:29], and so on.

I must leave to the philosophers debate as to the source of the sanctity of life and whether the principle can exist inside or outside of religion — or in both spheres. Such questions are beyond my field of competence. But it seems that what Mr. Callahan has to say is relevant to a number of areas which are of keen interest to me. I might mention one or two examples.

There have been, as anyone interested in the field knows, arguments and charges, sometimes bitter, concerning various aspects of human experimentation. In all of this welter a clear issue can be seen emerging. It is above personalities; it is above legalistics; it is simply this: in experimentation with man is the individual subject to get first consideration or does this belong to society? It is time the debate was directed to this fundamental issue.

Society certainly has rights, recognized in law and by all men of good will, in the invasion of the individual's privacy by the census; in the legal requirement of certain standards of education and of hygiene, in the required reporting of venereal disease, in vaccination, in maintenance of civil order, in the required acceptance of the military draft (in war time a life-or-death issue).

It is evident that at times society properly acts against the wishes of the individual and without his consent. Thus, while freedom of choice, of consent, must stand very high, the freedom is not total as illustrated in the examples just mentioned. At times the decision has to be made against the individual to protect society. This is a grave and central problem.

Notwithstanding these and other exceptions where society must come first, there are, it seems to me, cogent reasons why *as a general principle* the individual must have priority in human experimentation. We shall examine these reasons in the hope that advocates for the preeminence of society will also tackle this complex problem and attempt to substantiate it from *their* point of view.

A healthy society requires healthy treatment of individuals. A truly divisive debate on this theme has been going on like an iceberg, seven-eighths below the surface, one-eighth above.

Unfortunately, those who opt for society, "the most good for the most people" as they say (sometimes in justification for their free-wheeling experimentation) have scornfully tagged those who believe in the supremacy of the individual as "zealots," "one-track zealots," "zealous crusaders," "extremists," and so on. The descent into name calling is regrettable. So far, those who choose "the greatest good for the greatest number" have had their derisive say; the other side has not chosen to reply in kind. But they could.

The "zealots" have unfortunately annoyed the others who take, in their God-like view, the right to choose martyrs for science (Kety's phrase). In such acts, far more than annoyance is involved: they have a terrifying potential to harm progress in medicine.

In the hospital, decisions are constantly being made whereby some lives are saved and others lost. The control of these decisions is the issue and, where research is involved, it becomes particularly difficult to be certain of one's judgments. While society has a direct oversight of such decisions through a hospital's committee on research and in its committee on ethics, such groups nevertheless usually place greater emphasis on safety for present lives than on the welfare of masses of future lives (society). The wish of the individual cannot be the controlling element in deciding which life will be saved, which lost. The interests of society as well as the interests of the individual must figure in this; the question is which should get first consideration. In research, the more the risking of lives is official (societal) the more important the valid consent of the subject becomes. He must not be pressed, coerced, or tricked into a collaboration he would reject if fully informed.

As Calabresi has put it, we want a decision which reflects a societal choice and society's control over when subjects are to be risked for the common good; but at the same time, we do not want society to lose its role as the protector of individual lives [3]. These are conflicting desires, but both are essential to a decent society. In clinical investigation the physician has the power to determine which shall prevail at a given time, but an unanswered question is, does he have the right to make this choice? A rigid and pedantic following of customs, rules, codes, and laws could easily lead to the untenable conclusion that the supreme public interest is only that of society; exceptions must predominate. This is false; the individual has rights too, and these, barring a few exceptions, must predominate.

> Consent, though very useful in preserving the appearance that society hardly ever condones the sacrifice of an individual against his will, is unlikely to suffice where a too obvious societal choice to take victims is involved. . . . Even more important, consent cannot serve as the general control item which determines when the future good requires the taking of present lives. Therefore, it is to the development of a workable but not too obvious control system which can use various forms of consent as an adjunct that scholars seriously concerned with the problem of saving future lives and at the same time not undermining our commitment to the sanctity of individual present lives ought to be devoting themselves [3].

The close relationship of these matters to "statistical" morality is evident.

At the Dartmouth conference on "The Great Issues of Conscience in Modern Medicine," Warren Weaver described statistical morality as derived from "the prejudice against even permitting any one known specific individual to sacrifice his life for the common good," and yet "we have to, in a great many circumstances, submit a lot of individuals to a partial risk" with the result that even though "the risk is only one in a million, when a million are involved, one man will be dead with our acquiescence. . . . It is a comfort to our conscience that we don't know *where* it occurred or *when* it occurred. But that individual is just as dead as though we knew all about it" [8:4]. In such deep waters we strive for balance, but sometimes emerge with little more than questions and tangled arguments.

For example, in discussing new and uncertain risk against probable benefit, Lord Adrian spoke of the rise in Britain of mass radiography of the chest [1]. Four and a half million examinations were made in 1957. It has been calculated that bone marrow effects of the radiation might possibly have added as many as 20 cases of leukemia in that year; yet the examinations revealed 18,000 cases of pulmonary tuberculosis needing supervision, as well as thousands of other abnormalities. The 20 deaths from leukemia were only a remote possibility, but, Lord Adrian asks, if they were a certainty would they have been too high a price to pay for the early detection of tuberculosis in 18,000 people?

When the consideration is a faceless number in jeopardy, even if that number is known to be large, the matter is often treated with indifference, but if the situation involves a specific man trapped in a coal mine, no cost or effort is spared to rescue him, for "We know the man trapped in a coal mine, just as we often know the patient subjected to experimentation; the statistical accident victim we do not know — so we can ignore him" [3]. Thoughtful people must have known for a long time that health and life are sometimes lost in medical experimentation, but very little was said publicly about the matter. It was only when 22 specific, sick, elderly Jews had live cancer cells injected into them without their knowledge [6] and when Beecher [2] at about the same time, quite by coincidence, presented his 10 year study of ethics in medical experimentation, where specific examples were given, that a considerable public furor occurred. No such result was present in the preceding decade when Beecher not infrequently spoke and wrote in general terms on the same subject. The somewhat extreme reactions of praise by some and condemnation by others occurred only when he dealt with specific examples.

To return to Calabresi's analysis of the situation: there appears to be "a deep conflict between our fundamental need constantly to reaffirm our belief in the sanctity of life, and our practical placing of some values (including future lives) above an individual life" [3]. How can we resolve this conflict? Several factors must be incorporated into any satisfactory resolution. These can be suggested tentatively: Man is not very much interested in mankind in general; one cannot relate to many people, but one can identify himself with a single individual. Another quite different ingredient in any understanding of the problem surely is the fact that accidents are the result of chance, carelessness, or factors beyond control (the unseen crack in the axle), whereas human experimentation involves risk deliberately taken.

The extraordinary preoccupation of individuals and groups with "codes" looks like an attempt to place on society the responsibility for what may happen during human experimentation. If these "guides" are accepted by society and if the individual experimenter has followed them, then if an accident occurs the responsibility is not the investigator's, at least not his alone, but society's. Man is not willing to take the responsibility for mankind in the mass, only for individuals, yet, rather unfairly, he expects mankind, society, to protect him! One difficulty in all of this is that the individual experimenter cannot know how much risk society wants him to take for future benefit, but consultation with his peers can provide some help.

Society is the protector of individuals, but society must also maintain control over situations which inevitably lead to the sacrifice of some for the common good. Consider the decisions made during operation of the artificial kidney. The widow whose children are educated and grown will be rejected by society's committee in favor of the father of several young children. The widow will be allowed to die and the other saved by dialysis. It is more comfortable to look at this from a positive approach: Society has saved the young father rather than that it has sacrificed the widow; life has been sustained. The situation is different when specific lives are jeopardized or sacrificed as in the examples described by Beecher [2] on questionably ethical or unethical human experimentation with no immediate gain for a specific individual. In this case the gain is for faceless mankind in the future and the bystander is disquieted.

There is some quiet opposition to respect for the patient's rights, more than a casual observer might suppose. Not long ago a distinguished scientist said, with some heat, "The individual is not infinitely valuable." This clashes with Guttentag's (and my own) view: ". . . the use of force is not justified on a single person, even if millions of other lives could be saved by such an act. [One realizes] the act would not just save millions of lives but that, as an amoral act from the standpoint of democratic brotherhood, it might create millions of amoral sequels, and that the moral history of mankind is more important than the scientific" [5]. The act also clashes with Reston's view, "If there has been a decline of decency in the modern world and a revolt against law and fair dealing, it is precisely because of the decline in the belief in each man as something precious" [7].

REFERENCES

1. Adrian, E D: Priorities in medical responsibility, *Proceedings of the Royal Society of Medicine*, vol 56, 1963, pp 523–528.
2. Beecher, Henry K: Ethics and Clinical Research, *The New England Journal of Medicine*, vol 274, 1966, pp 1354–1360.
3. Calabresi, G: Reflections on Medical Experimentation on Humans, Conference on Ethical Aspects of Experimentation on Human Subjects, American Academy of Arts and Sciences, Boston, Massachusetts, Nov 3–4, 1967.
4. Cooley, T M: *A Treatise on the Law of Torts* (Callaghan, Chicago, Illinois) 1888.
5. Guttentag, O E: The Problem of Experimentation on Human Beings. II. The Physician's Point of View, *Science*, vol 117, 1953, pp 207–210.
6. Langer, E: Human Experimentation: Cancer Studies at Sloan-Kettering Stir Public Debate on Medical Ethics, *Science*, vol 143, 1964, pp 551–553.
7. Reston, James: Washington: The Capital and the Easter Story, *The New York Times*, Apr 18, 1965.
8. Weaver, Warren: The Problem of Statistical Morality, *The Dartmouth Alumni Magazine Supplement*, November 1960.

RESPONSE

by Daniel Callahan

M ORE THAN IS OFTEN the case in such exercises of criticism, I find the comments on my article helpful and provocative. They pushed me along and I hope will do the same for the reader. I would like to respond principally to Professor Gustafson's remarks. I do so not because they necessarily raise issues more difficult and grave than those of Dr. Beecher and Dr. Pleasants, but mainly because I can in the context they provide also deal in some unified fashion with all of the comments.

The first theoretical question Professor Gustafson in effect puts to me is this: What are the ultimate justifications for the normative principles embodying a valuation of the sanctity of life, and what difference do different kinds of ultimate justifications make when judgments are made in particular cases? My response to the first part of the question must be brief. I think the "ultimate justifications" for any final, ultimate normative principles must be human experience. But since human experience does not, by itself, deliver principles, it is always necessary to have some kind of metaphysical principles to interpret and organize experience. The most pressing difficulties rarely arise over what experience actually delivers, though these difficulties should not be minimized. The critical problems more often turn on the meaning and implications of different kinds of experiences; thus are we pushed back to our ultimate metaphysical insights, affirmations, and perspectives.

The most critical problem of all, it seems to me, is what we choose to count as "ultimate" and how we go about justifying our choice. My own essential position is that the ultimate justification of normative principles rests upon their capacity to serve two functions. First, they show themselves to be coherent with our entire reading of the nature of things; they make sense in terms of our metaphysics. Second, they seem to us to be borne out in our lived experience, producing moral progress, sensitivity, and perceptiveness. Now I think it evident, (to leave aside the essential and perhaps inherent vagueness of these two norms of justification), that "ultimate justifications" will always, in an important sense, be circular. The logical conundrum here is that it is always necessary to justify any "ultimate justification" as indeed "ultimate"; that process inevitably seems to mean the introduction of an endless series of further, or deeper, presuppositions, each in turn requiring a justification of its own. I think, in the end, we are almost forced to break through this circularity (in practice, if not in theory) by an existential choice. We decide, for reasons both rational and a-rational, that we can push the issue no further and that we have reached a point of diminishing insight; at that stage, we choose our final (or first) starting point, hoping that it will express and affirm all that our limited wisdom has been able to conclude.

In the second part of the question, bearing on the difference which different kinds of ultimate justifications make for practical judgments, a number of issues need to be sorted out. There is, I believe, the empirical question whether in fact ultimate moral justifications resting on a religious basis (e.g., Christian or Jewish or Hindu) lead to significantly different moral decisions, practices, and mores than those resting on a non-religious basis. As one might expect, this question has a long and confusing history. I think it has been the working assumption of the adherents of most of the important religious traditions that these traditions do or should lead to moral decisions and practices discernibly different from those exhibited by the non-religious. The difficulties with this assumption, however, are notorious: professed believers often act as badly as professed non-believers, and professed non-believers often act in ways identical with (and as good as) the way in which believers act. The impact of this observation has, of late, led some believers to wonder whether the possession of an ultimate religious justification does in fact make any significant difference in the way people actually behave; Anthony Levi and Michael Novak have both argued recently that it does not, or is at least not the most significant variable in determining moral behavior. They are both most persuasive on this point, though neither has, in my opinion, taken sufficient account of the possibility that those non-religious men they single out as "good" are so singled out because their behavior happens to coincide with an implicit Judeo-Christian norm. It has, in any event, proved very difficult to empirically show that the moral behavior of the "average" believer can be predicted with certainty from a knowledge merely of that believer's professed religious perspective and commitment. It is this lack of predictability which has provided opponents of religion with so much material for the charge of hypocrisy; the same lack has provided religious "prophets" (in the Old Testament sense) with a fertile ground for righteous condemnation of what passes for religion.

Another issue to be sorted out bears on the more specific question of whether religious beliefs function to establish limits, particularly limits to "man's tampering with human life." My own impression is that the establishment of limits has been one of the most important thrusts of religion, particularly in its Judaic and Christian forms. Traditionally, Jewish, Protestant, and Catholic theologians had little difficulty agreeing that man's life is not entirely in his own hands, either individually or collectively (the quotations I provided in my essay from Karl Barth, Paul Ramsey, and Norman St. John-Stevas on stewardship are as "orthodox" as any could be). And the assumption underlying this tendency to set limits directly stems from the fundamental belief in a "transcendent" God, a God who provides and grounds values, norms, and laws (just which and how is of course hotly argued) which man, for his own good, is obliged to recognize. Correlatively, it has frequently been contended that a society which recognizes those limits stemming from a divine rather than a human source will be, all things equal, a safer, more secure society for its inhabitants. For it will not then be open to individuals or majorities capriciously and subjectively to make or break the recognized limits.

Two problems arise here. One is whether such societies have provided more security. This may perhaps be doubted since most mass religious societies have found ways to justify war, capital punishment, and abortion. Yet such societies have also possessed an ideal of human limits which, so they believe, generally works for the protection of life. Another problem is whether it is really of the essence of a religious ethic to be an ethic of limits and boundaries. At present, Christian ethics is being heavily influenced by variant forms of situation ethics, most of which would agree that whatever Christian ethics is, it is best not thought of as an ethics of law. More generally, Christian theology is being influenced by the pervasive idea that perhaps God left man considerably more freedom to work out his own destiny and values (including control over life and death) than was granted by traditional theology. Hence, while it might be possible to say safely that past Christian theology did have the function of setting firm limits to tampering with human life, this may not be the case much longer. I myself welcome this development since, as indicated in my essay, I think the protection actually offered human life in religious cultures has often been more theoretical than actual.

This last problem touches upon Professor Gustafson's concluding series of questions. I feel certain that the present confusion about the reverence for life is very directly related to a growing, worldwide secularization. On the one hand, this secularization has meant that men increasingly believe and feel that they are masters of their destiny, including the control of their own human life. Whether there is actually a loss of the sense of the transcendent is uncertain, but there seems to me decidedly a loss of the sense that somehow the transcendent by its very nature imposes fixed limits to human decisions and directions. On the other hand, secularization has meant the flourishing of pluralistic value systems, an important consequence of which is to relativize all of them. Or, more precisely, as Peter Berger has contended brilliantly in *The Sacred Canopy*, pluralism seems to rob religious and value systems of their self-evident, "factual" quality; they are then perceived to be matters of faith and belief rather than simply "the way things are." Thus it is one thing for men to reverence life because they think, as a simple matter of indubitable, accessible fact, that God requires this of them, and quite another because they believe their own particularistic, disputable religious faith implies such reverence.

I have no doubt that a subjective respect for life is easier to sustain when men believe, as a matter of objective fact, that God requires respect for life. But, as suggested earlier, the possibility that societies which did possess that belief were not really so protective of life in practice as their defenders would like to imagine raises the question whether the most important component in the actual (rather than hoped-for) respect accorded life is the religious element. It may well be that an ultimate religious justification of a moral principle is not, taken by itself, at all sufficient to condition attitudes and dispositions favorably to respect for life. My own guess, heeding the psychologists, is that a childhood nurturing strong on affection, love, and care is the most important conditioning element. Of course it may be that the context for this kind of nurture would best be a religious context; one could start a good brawl with that proposition. One way or the other, though, I think that Professor Gustafson is absolutely right in saying that if we are reduced to attending "only to the rational bases for making moral judgments," we are a long way from winning the game.

"Motivational energy," Professor Pleasants' phrase, has an important bearing here. It is doubtful on something as fundamental as respect for life whether reasoning, reading, writing, and final rational consensus could ever provide a deep enough respect to carry the majority of mankind through moments of crisis. All societies and all nations, so far as I know, pay lip service to the need to respect life; yet that just doesn't seem to stop the killing, the wars, and all the immoralities which violate human dignity. What is lacking seems to be a thoroughly deep-seated rational and emotional repugnance in the face of a temptation to violate life. National, private, and scientific "interests" have a way of washing principles away or enabling us to rationalize their meaning in a way favorable to our interests. Dr. Pleasants makes an important point in stressing the impersonality of modern methods of killing; they very effectively help circumvent the repugnance which the taking of life arouses. In my more apocalyptic moments, I am sometimes prone to think that only a major technological disaster — a nuclear war would do — could make human beings sufficiently sensitive to the hazards of *seemingly* impersonal methods of death and degradation. But I hope a less costly way can be found to achieve the same ends. We need, as a human community, an ethical imagination backed by an effective impulse of great power to provide a sufficiently safe human environment.

Dr. Beecher points to a number of medical dilemmas relevant to Dr. Pleasants' concern with impersonality and also relevant to Professor Gustafson's observation that the language of "rights" carries a different accent than the language of "value." Up to a point, Professor Gustafson is undoubtedly correct. It is less easy, for instance, to defend the "value" of the individual than the "value" of the common good; the individual has much going against him when his value is weighed on a scale overbalanced by the collective value of all individuals. It would seem, then, that the language of "rights," especially "inalienable rights," provides the individual with greater protection; it takes him off the scale altogether. A major complication, however, is that many current medical problems have been couched in the language of "rights," with almost as much confusion and uncertainty as that engendered by talk of "value." The abortion debate has seen the putative "right of women" not to have an "unwanted child" brought into conflict with the "right to life" of the fetus, and it is easy to imagine the conflicts Dr. Beecher points to couched as a conflict of rights: the "right to life" of present individuals in conflict with the collective "right to life" of many as yet unborn individuals. Another complication is that the language of rights is most effective in establishing limits when there is a consensus on the hierarchical order of rights, e.g., that the "right to life" takes precedence over all other rights. But as we know it is not easy to gain agreement on the proper hierarchical order. The most serious complication, however, can be put in the form of a question: Is the language of rights an irreducible, non-translatable language or does it presuppose an underlying affirmation of values? Phrased differently, does a system of claimed "rights" depend upon a prior system of values or is it *sui generis?* I must confess that I don't know the answer to these questions. But my own suspicion is that much would depend upon the particular ethical system in question; some, conceivably, would permit a translation of "rights" into "values" or a derivation of the former from the latter, while others might not. It would not, in any case, seem to me logically impermissible for someone to ask, upon hearing the phrase "right to life," what "value" this right is meant to serve; it would have to be shown that the language of "rights" has a status more primitive or fundamental than the language of "values."

Finally, a word on "generalizability." Obviously there is a connection between Professor Gustafson's concerns here and the point touched upon by Dr. Beecher at the end of his comment. Beecher's quote from Guttentag, which expresses a worry about "amoral sequels," seems to me another and more concrete way of discussing the issue of "generalizability." Or is it? To return to where we started, one of the contentions of the "religious" viewpoint (e.g., those of Ramsey and St. John-Stevas) is that it provides protection because it takes certain decisions of life and death out of human hands; no calculations of relative value and utility are allowed. One does not, in a word, have to even try to answer the question "what would happen if everyone did that?" That is a good question, to be sure, but the thrust of the religious grounding of values (at least pushed in a fundamentalist direction) is that the very asking of such a question opens the way for placing human life in jeopardy. For who could know in advance, under all circumstances, what the answer might be? Could it not happen that in a context of desperate poverty a decision to give all parents the right to kill all infants would seem a wise one? The religious viewpoint, by refusing to recognize certain questions as valid, is intent on avoiding all questions whose answers may be uncertain in a calculus of relative values or rights. It wants certain acts judged wrong even if there is no possibility of proving that "amoral sequels" will follow. The great difference, then, between a religious and a non-religious foundation for normative principles (to oversimplify) would seem to be that the former would place final calculations in the hands of God while the latter would believe that they must be made by humans. I believe, though, that the former position is no longer tenable; it is the latter which must now be given a "religious" foundation and corrective.

9. TWO MODERN DOCTRINES OF NATURE

by Frederick Elder

In our day of exponential human population growth, multiform environmental pollution and ever-expanding urban perimeters, not to mention heart transplants, space probes, and the synthesis of elemental life forms, the doctrine of nature has begun to re-emerge as an item of more than passing theological interest. Modern man finds himself as the possessor of both unprecedented power and a growing feeling of helplessness, and in this condition he asks critical questions, some of which fall under the rubric of a doctrine of nature. Among the relevant questions are ones such as these: What is man in relation to nature, a being apart from the given environment or one inextricably bound up with it? What is the proper position concerning the issue of control, i.e., control of nature by man and control of man by nature? What, indeed, is the proper response to the natural order based not only on considerations of control but also on considerations of what the natural order is per se?

I want to present here two contemporary doctrines of nature which go about answering such questions in strikingly different ways. The first of these comes from a man who is not a professed religionist, Loren Eiseley, Benjamin Franklin Professor of Anthropology and the History of Science at the University of Pennsylvania. He writes as a scientist, and his work exhibits the empirical exactness that is expected of a man of science. Yet the prose of this scientist also reveals an aesthetic dimension as well as a discernment which can be described only as religious. His is not a doctrinal religion, and yet the rudiments of at least a doctrine of nature are clearly evident in his work.

The second doctrine of nature is taken from a triumvirate of modern Christian thinkers. Two of these are Protestant theologians, Harvey Cox and Herbert Richardson; the third is Teilhard de Chardin, the late Jesuit paleontologist. I have chosen these three particular men because I think they exhibit remarkable similarities in their doctrines of nature. Their expressions of the doctrine certainly differ, but the essential elements in them are the same. Another reason for choosing them is because each one has been recognized as a venturesome writer and thus is considered by many as being in the very forefront of imaginative Christian writing. Finally, these three, if their kind of view is accepted, absolutely obviate the kind of view held by Eiseley and thus represent the sharpest theological contrast it is possible to draw in regard to this particular doctrine.

MAN AND NATURE

Turning to the first question posed above, i.e., what is man's relation to nature? we find that the anthropologist Eiseley, pre-eminently an evolutionist, gives an answer that can be described as biocentric. In company with many of his fellow life scientists, he sees all life on earth in a state of interrelatedness, of symbiotic "complementation." Life is seen as a gestalt, with the whole understood as greater than the sum of its parts. Therefore, it is an error to ever isolate man from the rest of nature and treat him as though he were the only center of value. To Eiseley man is a wonder, but man is not the only wonder or possibly even the last one. As he puts it:

> In many a fin and reptile foot I have seen myself passing by — some part of myself, that is, some part that lies unrealized in the momentary shape I inhabit. People have written me harsh letters and castigated me for a lack of faith in man when I have ventured to speak of this matter in print. . . . They would bring God into the compass of a shopkeeper's understanding and confine him to these limits, lest He proceed to some unimaginable and shocking act — create, perhaps as a casual afterthought, a being more beautiful than man. As for me, I believe nature capable of this, and . . . I feel no envy — any more than

the frog envies the reptile or an ancestral ape should envy man
[11:24–25].

In Eiseley's view the trouble stems from what he calls man's
continuing Ptolemaic vision. Man sees himself as the culmination
and the end. If man were to cease to be, it is felt that the sun
would go out and the earth blacken. Everything that lives apart
from man is seen as having only a contingent worth, dependent
on what it can be or do for man. Against this, he sees the value
of life, in whatever form, as intrinsic.

In contradistinction we may notice what our trio of Christian
writers say. Chardin, who, interestingly enough, shared the evo-
lutionary point of view of Eiseley, chose, nevertheless, to put
a completely different stress upon it. Where Eiseley places value
on the whole process of life, viewing it as a web out of which
come many emergents, Chardin narrowed his perspective down
to just one emergent — the one he considered the last — man. As
he said in the preface to *The Phenomenon of Man*, "I have
chosen man as the center, and around him I have tried to establish a coherent order between antecedents and consequents"
[4:29].

Now Chardin presents himself as an objective scientist in his
writing, but why he chose man as the center of his investigation
stems, I suggest, from his implicit understanding of Creation as
that manifested in the dominant Christian view. That view becomes much more explicit in Cox and Richardson, both of whom
turn to the major seedbed of the Christian concept of man and
nature, the biblical Creation narratives. Cox leans heavily on the
Yahwistic account of Creation in Genesis, claiming that the
"Hebrew view of Creation . . . separates nature from God and
distinguishes man from nature" [8:22]. Elsewhere, again with
emphasis on the Yahwistic narrative plus Genesis 1:28, the famous "dominion" verse of the priestly account of Creation, he
states that "God does not simply insert man into a world filled
with creatures which are already named, in relationships already
established by decree. Man must fashion them himself. He simply
doesn't discover meaning; he originates it [8:74]. In the Yahwistic

account man is created first and other creatures follow, obtaining their names — their identity — from man. As a result, man has both "priority rights" in Creation and is the sole arbiter of the fate of the rest of it. Cox's view, then, is clearly anthropocentric, putting him in full accord with Chardin.

Anthropocentrism is the dominant theme in Richardson, also, though he concentrates on the priestly account of Creation as his justifying source. Noting that the priestly narrative places man last in the order of Creation, he claims that this is a literary device designed to show that what comes later in the order is to be of higher significance. "Man as the last creature formed by God," he claims, "is also the highest creature; to him is given the right of dominion over every other created thing. All other creatures are less than man from the point of view of what is technically called 'dignity'; they are all created for his sake and ordered to his good" [18:115–116].

Our three Christian writers thus are strongly anthropocentric with regard to man's relation to nature. They stand in sharp opposition to Eiseley's biocentric view which sees man as one center among many. In their adherence to this position these venturesome writers turn out to be remarkably orthodox. For as an historian wrote,

> Especially in its Western form, Christianity is the most anthropocentric religion the world has seen. As early as the 2nd century both Tertullian and Saint Irenaeus of Lyon were insisting that when God shaped Adam he was foreshadowing the image of the incarnate Christ, the Second Adam. Man shares, in great measure, God's transcendence of nature. Christianity, in absolute contrast to ancient paganism and Asia's religions (except, perhaps, Zoroastrianism) not only established a dualism of man and nature but also insisted that it is God's will that man exploit nature for his proper ends [25].

With the contrasting anthropocentric and biocentric views now taken as the basic presuppositions, I turn to see how the next question which was posed, the one concerning the proper expression of control, is answered by the two doctrines.

CONTROL

Each of the "anthropocentrists" has a unique answer to this question, and yet each amounts to the same thing: man, in his position of absolute suzerainty upon earth, is to practice control of nature to a complete degree. Now, to be sure, they do not say this in just those words, yet what they each envision for the future, generally with approval, amounts to just that.

So it is that Cox sees nature completely subjugated by man's greatest expression of separation from the natural order, the city. "Future historians will record the twentieth century," he says, "as that century in which the whole world became one immense city" [7:101]. He elaborates by noting that "whereas [cities] once formed mere islands in a vast sea of uncharted nature, today the balance is reversing itself. The world is becoming one huge interdependent city, in which jungles and deserts remain only with the explicit consent of a global metropolis" [7:102]. Looking at the prospect of planetary urbanization the theologian's reaction is recorded when he says, "It is thrilling to live in the age of the new world city . . ." [7:102].

In Richardson's view nature's subjugation will seemingly be complete, since he foresees "the creation of a wholly artificial environment" [18:17]. Such an environment will be the product of a proliferating "sociotechnics," by which he means the increasing conjunction of man and machine. This conjunction will not be in the form of man controlling machines as is the common view, or, somehow, machines controlling men on the same subject-object basis as the other; rather, men and machines will actually control one another on a "continuing cycle of inquiry and feedback" [18:18]. With sociotechnics, "an entire society will organize in order to reshape itself and its world in accordance with an imaginative vision of the good life" [18:17], rather than follow the previous practice of using nature as a pattern in the art of control. Thus man's control will be absolute and in the midst of the wholly artificial environment the given systems will, seemingly, cease to exist.

Chardin's anthropocentric vision of the future concentrates on the now-famous noosphere or layer of thought, if you please, which is now being formed "above" the virtually conquered biosphere, the natural systems layer. This noosphere is "a single organized membrane over the earth" [4:164], where man with his facilities of travel and communications is in a state of forming "an almost solid mass of hominized substance" [4:240]. "Hominization" is the process whereby man becomes truly human as he achieves perfect unity in diversity among human kind, so that man actually becomes a single psycho-social unit, an organism, that will finally reach a terminal transcendent point, Omega, which he sometimes links with God.

In moving toward the transcendent stage, man, to put it bluntly, crunches nature by means of science and technology. Chardin himself puts it more elegantly, saying, "Taken in the full modern sense of the word, science is the twin sister of mankind," for, "the march of humanity develops indubitably in the direction of a conquest of matter put to the service of mind" [4:248–249]. His view is that all nature longs to be mankind and that the earth realizes its ultimate worth only when the unit, man, comes to full expression. Proper control means promoting the process of making nature into mankind.

Eiseley, on the other hand, viewing life within a biocentric context, holds that control does *not* completely reside in man. He does not for a minute deny man's manipulative capacity or his mental ability to transcend the natural order by means of art, imagination, and spiritual awareness. But he dwells on the fact that man is a biological organism and as such is subject to biological laws. "If we get too remote," he warns, "from the world out of which we came — too remote from green leaves, too remote from waters, ancestral waters in the sense that we carry [them] in our living bodies — there is a danger that in the mechanical constructions which the mind itself can create that we may forget that we exist and live by this world out of which we have emerged" [10]. Eiseley elaborates on this, relating it specifically to the contemporary era this way:

One might say that all organisms that run loose, that escape for the moment out of the living web that controls them, have this potential danger within them. If one flies over any extended area of the country I think that one can almost see this as one might look at fungus spreading on an orange. Because one sees these great urban concentrations of people spreading and spreading, the forest disappearing, the concrete highways extending farther and farther, and although in a sense, and momentarily perhaps, it represents the spread of civilization, along with it goes this danger of overpopulation, this divorce once again from the nature that we are far more dependent [upon] than we realize [10].

The scientist considers general ecological factors which heretofore were not of primary importance, when neither man's numbers filled the earth nor his technology was able to drastically alter the balance of nature. Now he says they are of such importance and, indeed, are ultimately determinant. It is these very factors which the "anthropocentrists," conditioned to think within a narrower context, generally ignore.

[It is true that toward the end of his book [4] Chardin does seem to take ecological factors into consideration. Everything prior to page 283 has emphasized man's uniqueness and his control of the earth. But on that page he abruptly mentions the need of a whole series of "geo-sciences," including geo-demography, as well as "the control of the trek toward unpopulated areas." This kind of emphasis means that he is suddenly talking about man not controlling nature as much as man controlling himself. And a control of the trek toward unpopulated areas is a statement that stands in sharp contrast to an "almost solid mass of hominized substance." I gain the impression that Chardin, almost as an afterthought, realizes that the inherent limitations of the earth have to be dealt with in a way other than simply characterizing them as forcing the "hominization" of man, the latter being produced by man's ever-increasing growth of population and invention. This section is an anomaly in the book, for its implications cast a shadow over the emphasis which is given everywhere else.]

Turning now to the last of our questions, we come to a consideration of what the proper response to the natural order is to be. In terms of control the answers of the two doctrines have already been given. Our Christian writers have said it is to be a response of power resulting in subjugation, even to the point of complete transformation of the given environment. Eiseley has indicated that in matters of control man must realize that ultimately he is the object of it more than he is its subject.

With respect to questions of response to nature beyond those dealt with under the heading of control the "anthropocentrists" have virtually nothing to say. Having already extracted man out of nature (Cox), or pictured him as either an all-encompassing final emergent (Chardin), or a culminating expression of nature who rightfully exerts complete dominance (Richardson), they leave the natural order (*sans manu*) as no more than the setting of man's activity as well as the raw material which he fashions into whatever form best pleases him. For them there is nothing in the non-human part of nature which indicates a non-contingent value, including religious value. Cox, for example, is most explicit at this point, emphasizing how the Christian faith has "desacralized" nature, stripping it of any status as a divine entity in and of itself and leaving it as no more than the object subject to man [8:24].

THE RELIGIOUS DIMENSION

It is precisely here that Eiseley's view contrasts most sharply with the other, and it is at this same point where the religious dimension of the anthropologist's awareness comes to full expression. Where our modern Christian writers have stripped nature of any separate, not to mention spiritual, significance, Eiseley sees in it significance of the highest order.

This scientist has a perception that stretches beyond the measurable (although that is important, especially ecologically), and beyond that which is merely pleasing to the senses. As he puts it, "I . . . want to look at this natural world both from the empirical point of view and from one which also takes into account that sense of awe and marvel which is a part of man's primitive heritage, and without which man would not be man." He goes on to add, "For many of us the Biblical bush still burns, and there is a deep mystery in the heart of a simple seed" [9:179].

Eiseley's view is preternatural, seeing the extraordinary in the ordinary, the uncommon in the common. Mood and setting and circumstance arouse in him an awareness that tells of something that is both strangely familiar and familiarly different. In a term given to us by Rudolf Otto, it can be said that Eiseley has an awareness of the numinous.

In one of the appendices to his book, *The Idea of the Holy*, Otto cites a passage from John Ruskin which the theologian describes as wholly numinous in character. It has to do with the natural order and reads like something out of Eiseley. Speaking of the perception of his youth Ruskin said:

> . . . there was a continual perception of Sanctity in the whole of nature, from the slightest to the vastest, an instinctive awe mixed with delight; an indefinable thrill, such as we sometimes imagine to indicate the presence of a disembodied spirit. I could only feel this perfectly when I was alone; and then it would often make me shiver from head to foot with the joy and fear of it, when after some time away from hills I first got to the shore of a mountain river . . . or when I first saw the swell of distant land against the sunset, or the first low broken wall, covered with mountain moss . . . the joy in nature seemed to me to come of a sort of heart-hunger, satisfied with the presence of a Great and Holy Spirit . . . [20:215].

Such a passage is like those offered in Eiseley; indeed, the literature of the anthropologist is replete with them. For the sake of illustration I shall quote one such passage *in toto* in order to give the full flavor of Eiseley's numinous experience. The following account comes from a time when he was on an archaeological expedition in the Badlands of the American West:

It was a late hour on a cold windbitten day when I climbed a great hill spine like a dinosaur's back and tried to take my bearings. The tumbled waste fell away in waves in all directions. Blue air was darkening into purple along the bases of the hills. I shifted my knapsack, heavy with the petrified bones of long-vanished creatures, and studied my compass. I wanted to be out of there by nightfall, and already the sun was going down suddenly in the west.

It was then that I saw the flight coming on. It was moving like a little close-knit body of black specks that danced and darted and closed again. It was pouring from the north and heading toward me with the undeviating relentlessness of a compass needle. It streamed through the shadows rising out of monstrous gorges. It rushed toward towering pinnacles in the red light of the sun, or momentarily sank from sight within their shade. Across the desert of eroding clay and wind-worn stone they came with a faint wild twittering that filled all the air about me as those tiny living bullets hurtled past into the night.

It may not strike you as a marvel. It would not perhaps unless you stood in the middle of a dead world at sunset, but that was where I stood. Fifty million years lay under my feet, fifty million years of bellowing monsters moving on in a green world now gone so utterly that its very light was travelling on the farther edge of space. The chemicals of all that vanished age lay about me in the ground. Around me lay the shearing molars of dead titanotheres, the delicate sabers of soft-stepping cats, the hollow sockets that had held the eyes of many a strange, outmoded beast. Those eyes had looked out upon a world as real as ours; dark, savage brains had roamed and roared their challenges into the steaming night.

Now they were still there, or, put it as you will, the chemicals that made them were here about me in the ground. The carbon that had driven them ran blackly in the eroding stone. The stain of iron was in the clays. The iron did not remember the blood it had once moved within, the phosphorus had forgot the savage brain. The little individual moment had ebbed from all those strange combinations of chemicals as it would ebb from our living bodies into the sinks and runnels of oncoming time.

I had lifted up a fistful of that ground. I held it while that wild flight of southbound warblers hurtled over me into the oncoming darkness. There went phosphorus, there went iron, there went carbon, there beat the calcium in those hurrying wings. Alone on a dead planet I watched that incredible miracle speeding past. It ran by some true compass over field and waste land. It cried its individual ecstasies into the air until the gullies rang. It swerved like a single body, it knew itself and, lonely, it bunched close in the racing darkness, its individual entities feeling about them the rising night. And so, crying to each other their identity, they passed away out of my view.

I dropped my fistfull of earth. I heard it roll inanimate back into the gully at the base of the hill: iron, carbon, the chemicals of life. Like men from those wild tribes who had hunted these hills before me seeking visions, I made my sign to the great darkness. It was not a mocking sign, and I was not mocked. As I walked into my camp late that night, one man, rousing from his blankets beside the fire, asked sleepily, "What did you see?"

"I think a miracle," I said softly, but I said it to myself [11:172–173].

For Eiseley the world is an arena of miracles; the natural world in its entirety is a miracle. "We forget," he says, "that nature itself is one vast miracle transcending the reality of night and nothingness." And he goes on to add, significantly, "We forget that each one of us in his personal life repeats that miracle" [9:171]. Man is truly wondrous, but that is only because he is an expression of an order that in its entirety is wondrous. Moreover, the presence of the wondrous world implies the reality of a wonder-worker. "I would say," offers Eiseley, "that if 'dead' matter has reared up this curious landscape of fiddling crickets, song sparrows, and wondering men, it must be plain even to the most devoted materialist that the matter of which he speaks contains amazing, if not dreadful powers, and may not impossibly be, as Hardy has suggested, 'but one mask of many worn by the Great Face behind'" [11:210].

Eiseley is a living datum supporting the thesis of Otto, and he is a very important one since he is a learned scientist with his credentials fully in order and his renown rather widespread. He embodies and gives very eloquent expression to a consciousness that could be dismissed only if he were judged mentally unbalanced. And instead of that most of his critics have come away feeling that his consciousness has made modern man appear mentally deprived. His awareness is a direct challenge to those who would allot the whole value of Creation to *Homo sapiens*.

ECOLOGICAL DATA

With the contrasts between our two modern doctrines of nature now drawn, I would like to turn to a defense of the one I think more valid, the one advocated by Eiseley. To present a full defense it is necessary first to offer the relevant physical, i.e., ecological data. As noted previously, it is this kind of data which has been virtually ignored by the "anthropocentrists," primarily because they have not been trained to think in terms of the impact of specific acts of human endeavor upon the given systems of the natural environment. However, such data now strongly suggest that man in his various technological expressions, based on the anthropocentric view inherited from the dominant Christian attitude toward nature, is pushing toward the inherent limits of the earth, the violation of which will set off the most dire repercussions. Much of the world, of course, is not under specific Christian influence. Yet virtually the entire world has felt the effect of the technological revolution, and that had its origin and has its main expression in lands with Christianity in their background. In light of the kind of evidence which follows I would contend (1) that Eiseley is substantiated in his claim that man is ultimately more the object of control than its subject; and (2) that the "complete control" visions of our Christian writers, though imaginative presentations, are merely extensions of present trends which are now proving to be dangerous, and, if continued, will be disastrous.

1. Fundamental to all ecological considerations is the question of population. Viewing the earth as the biosphere one notes that one species is dominant, both in activity and numbers; that

species is *Homo sapiens*. It is increasing roughly at 2.0% per year [27], meaning that it will double its number in 35 years. Such an increase will put its 3.479 billion [27] at something near 7 billion shortly after the turn of the century. At present it is estimated that one billion persons are undernourished and an additional 800 million are deficient in one or more nutrients, so that more than half of humanity suffers from at least malnourishment [2:xi].

In ecological terms, any time a species in a defined area has insufficient food for half or more of its number it is considered in imbalance. This is exactly the circumstance of humanity on earth. Moreover, as the Special Task Force on Environmental Health reported to the Department of Health, Education and Welfare of the United States Government, "Virtually every assessment of environmental problems attributed them, in substantial measure, to the combined effects of increasing population (particularly urban population) and industrialization" [23:16]. Yet it is these twin causes of environmental problems which are taken for granted in Cox's view of the emerging world city and Chardin's "almost solid mass of hominized substance."

2. Turning to some of those problems arising from increasing human numbers and industrialization, I shall begin by looking at air pollution. Awareness of air pollution and some of its effects is now general among the informed public. It is well-known that it exacerbates the condition of those with respiratory diseases, generally dirties and on occasion corrodes surfaces within urban areas, and forms the familiar smog cloud which offends the aesthetic sense of at least some persons.

What may not be so well-known are the possible worldwide effects of air pollution and how they endanger mankind and all other forms of life. For example, there is the problem of the effect of carbon dioxide on the atmosphere. A summary of the situation is presented as follows:

> Carbon dioxide is being added to the earth's atmosphere by the burning of coal, oil and natural gas at the rate of 6 billion tons a year. By the year 2000 there will be about 25% more

CO_2 in our atmosphere than at present. This will modify the heat balance of the atmosphere to such an extent that marked changes in climate not controllable through local or even national efforts, could occur [17:9].

The overall result of increased carbon dioxide in the air is a general heating of the atmosphere. Calculating what could happen to the antarctic ice cap as a result of this heating, it is conceivable that the runoff could raise sea level some four feet every ten years, forty feet per century [17:123]. Needless to say, this would cause devastation to the coastal areas of the world.

Another aspect of air pollution may yield a situation whereby the problem is not an unwelcome addition to the atmosphere but a depletion of its vital property. As an editorial in *The Christian Century* put it:

> According to scientist Lamont C. Cole of Cornell University, the human community is in danger of running out of oxygen. Oxygen shortage has occasionally been shown to exist in the United States, Japan and Great Britain. Although the world-wide circulation of air, which is about 20 per cent oxygen, makes up for local shortages, it may not continue to do so unless some thought is given to conserving oxygen-producing vegetation. The chance sinking of a few tankers carrying plant poisons could seriously diminish the capacity of sea plants — the source of 70 per cent of the earth's oxygen — to supply this vital element. The destruction of rain forests by heedless industrialization could have the same effect. Professor Cole points out that the increase of human and animal population, the spread of fires and the destruction of greenery push us all toward the danger point [5].

The mention of the chance sinking of ships is not irrelevant. The break-up of oil-bearing ships in the oceans causing widespread oil pollution has become a recent tragedy of far too frequent occurrence. Such chance happenings point to a very important part of ecological considerations, the weak link aspect, which I shall discuss subsequently.

3. Pollution of the air is being matched if not exceeded by the pollution of water, at least in the industrialized countries. As in

other areas, the industrial leader, the United States, serves as the outstanding example.

Dr. Barry Commoner, citing a report to the Federal Council for Science and Technology by the Committee on Pollution in 1966, mentions that, "among other things the report points out that at the present rate of accumulation of pollutants, essentially all of the surface waters of the United States will become so contaminated as to lose their biological capability for purification within the next twenty years" [6:144n]. This is substantiated by Dr. Harold A. Thomas, Jr., of Harvard's School of Public Health and Center for Population Studies, who feels that by 1980 American streams and lakes will provide insufficient oxygen to stabilize biochemically all the organic wastes produced by the economy [24].

Of course, water is treated to make it fit for human consumption and other use, and with increasing pollution the demands for treatment increase. In connection with that it may be noted what the present condition of water treatment is. The Task Force on Environmental Health claimed that, "Fifty million Americans drink water that does not meet Public Health Service drinking water standards. Another 45,000,000 Americans drink water that has not been treated by the Public Health Service" [23:13]. Without strenuous efforts in the face of increased demands the situation, obviously, can only get worse.

4. Besides air and water pollution there is also the so-called "third pollutant," the solid waste accumulation, or trash. In America one billion square yards of trash are generated each year at present. Forty million old automobiles are rusting in junkyards or miscellaneous places. As of 1965, 4.5 pounds of solid waste were generated per person per day. If present trends continue the amount generated will be 18.0 pounds per person per day by A.D. 2000. And this, it is to be remembered, from a population that will be between one and a half and two times as large as it was in 1965 [13].

Not all solid waste, naturally, is kept in solid form. Some of it is buried, some is incinerated. Here, however, one appreciates interactions of different ecological problems. Burying of waste takes large amounts of land out of use, thus adding to the present problem of urban sprawl, while incineration adds to the problem of air pollution.

5. With the mention of interactions one touches upon what may be the most telling argument of those, such as Eiseley, who approach matters ecologically. They emphasize interactions and highlight the one which is unforeseen. I would characterize this as the "weak link" aspect of environmental situations. There are many examples.

First of all, dealing once again with the fundamental consideration of population, we note that after World War II worldwide public health measures were taken to promote increased death control, but that this effort was not accompanied by a balancing effort of birth control. As a result, human population skyrocketed and has now precipitated a desperate attempt to increase world food production and distribution. However, even if the desired increase in food production is achieved, the question remains as to what effect the new production will have on the earth's interrelated biological systems. In light of such things as the harmful effects of pesticides, the way fertilizers pollute natural water systems and the vulnerability of monoculture (one-crop) landscapes, it could be that solving the food problem will lead to the creation of even greater ecological problems. And this whole series of problems will have been set off by the unforeseen weak link of birth control.

Pesticides in and of themselves are a classic example of the weak link phenomenon. When they first came into use they were hailed as a panacea and widely used. They still are widely used, but in the interim doubts have been raised about their desirability. R. L. Rudd, who took up the work begun by Rachel Carson, would agree that pesticides have done some good but points to several different items which might be considered weak links in their usage. Some of these are:

1. Most pesticides are nonselective, i.e., they kill more than the intended victim or victims.

2. Their manner of use is often imprecise, i.e., they are broadcast over wide areas rather than carefully directed toward specific examples.

3. Many kinds of chemicals used (especially chlorinated hydrocarbons such as DDT) are stable and survive in soil, water and living tissue.

4. Many of the chemicals follow insidious routes such as those of delayed toxicity, secondary poisoning, etc. Thus the insecticides which kill, say, pests in a body of water may also kill fish which eat the pests as well as men who eat the fish [19:3–6, 43–56, 248–267].

Pesticides are an example of substances which were used before their full effect was even guessed. But pesticides hardly stand alone. "The Food and Drug Administration has estimated that the American people are being exposed to some 500,000 different substances, many of them over a long period of time. Yet fewer than ten per cent of these substances have been catalogued in a manner that might provide the basis for determining their effects on man and his environment" [23:5].

Another example of the weak link is given to us by an ecologist who touches upon the artificial society which looms so large in the thought of Richardson. He remarks how,

. . . there is good reason to believe that people could be conditioned to adjust themselves to a highly artificial technologically controlled environment such as the city under a plastic bubble which some envision. Such an arrangement, however, could not only congeal the pattern of living, but be vulnerable on two counts. The greater our dependence upon an elaborate chain of technology the more liable we become to disaster through failure of any link. And the more restricted our range of experience, even though physical needs are met, the greater our loss of flexibility to meet emergency. The too-sheltered child is an example. So is battery-grown poultry. These birds, raised under completely controlled conditions, must be protected against sudden noises or even the presence of a stranger. Otherwise they pile up in a corner and smother each other [22].

Such an account might be dismissed as reactionary if there were no examples to suggest that it might be true. But in fact such examples exist. In November, 1965, all the electric power in an 80,000 square mile area of the northeastern United States and Canada failed. The incident which triggered the entire blackout was the failure of one relay which led into a feeder line in one small part of the vast electrical network covering the affected area. The blackout was something which simply was not supposed to happen. It did. Speaking of the incident, Commoner notes that, "although the 'cause' of the blackout has been discovered in the sense that the failure began with the opening of an incorrectly set relay at Queenston, Ontario, the crucial point is that no one yet knows why that failure precipitated the spreading disaster. In other words, the power network was established before anyone understood the circumstances under which it would fail" [6:135n].

Another kind of artificial power network one can think of is the blanket of aircraft and submarines carrying nuclear weapons throughout the world. Here, too, is a system that is not supposed to fail. Yet in the last few years planes carrying these weapons have been lost on two different occasions. Fortunately no explosions ensued, and the world hopes that the third time is not the charm.

Other pertinent areas of concern could be cited in detail, among them the continuing diminution of the earth's forests, the steady extirpation of animal taxa, the effect of radioactivity and the possible effects of human overcrowding. However, I believe enough has been shown to adequately defend Eiseley and his biocentric position, at least as far as empirical data are concerned. Certainly many life scientists are extremely concerned and feel that a continuance of present trends forebodes nothing but evil. Their view was well expressed by Dr. Donald M. Gates, director of the Missouri Botanical Gardens, as he testified before a House subcommittee on science and technology. Dr. Gates said, "We do not understand the dynamics of a forest, grassland, ocean, lake, pond or river, nor are we proceeding rapidly enough toward this understanding. We will go down in history as an elegant technological society struck down by biological disintegration for lack of ecological understanding" [12].

THEOLOGICAL CONSIDERATIONS

My defense of Eiseley's position now moves into the area more familiar to most of the "anthropocentrists" — that of biblical material as well as Christian theology and history.

Turning first to Eiseley's biocentric emphasis, I would focus on the Creation narratives, which have had so much influence. Let it be acknowledged that the earlier, more primitive story, that of the Yahwist, which extends from Genesis 2:4 through the third chapter, is clearly not biocentric. Speaking of the emphasis of this narrative Gerhard von Rad says, "It is man's world, the world of his life (the sown, the garden, the animals, the woman), which God in what follows establishes *around man;* and this forms the primary theme of the entire narrative, 'adāmadāmā (man-earth). . . .' In this world, which is regarded quite anthropocentrically, man is the first creature" [16:74–75].

However, this account is only a half of the Creation "witness." The other view, the priestly account, which is given from Genesis 1 through 2:3, does not start with man but lists the order of Creation this way: vegetation, animals, man. Quite significantly, *each* of these is seen as good, and the fish and birds are specifically directed to multiply just as man is, with, I think, the implication being that multiplication applies to all forms of life. Man, to be sure, is given dominion (Genesis 1:28), but there seems to be no necessary command in this "commission" to diminish or destroy what has been created previously and pronounced good. Moreover, this narrative has God, not man, as the center of focus. This theocentric view speaks not only of earth but also of the heavens, indeed all that is, as traceable to the creating hand of God.

Now it is true that the priestly narrative is not as old as its counterpart, but this very fact might illustrate its greater sophistication and more trenchant view. From such a view the biocentric position can be defended. Without denying that man has suzerainty and a right to use the earth, it can be claimed that the earth has meaning apart from man (Richardson notwithstanding), because God has called it good even before man was present, and further, that use must be very carefully differentiated from abuse.

Such an interpretation would not be entirely new, nor one coming only from those outside Christian circles. For instance, C. F. D. Moule, the English theologian, takes exactly such a stance in his book, *Man and Nature in the New Testament,* which has the interesting subtitle: Some Reflections on Biblical Ecology. Moule interprets the *imago Dei* and man's dominion in terms of responsibility and stewardship, and summarizes his view by saying,

> Man is placed in the world by God to be its Lord. He is meant to have dominion over it and to use it . . . but only for God's sake, only like Adam in paradise, cultivating it for the Lord. As soon as he begins to use it selfishly, and reaches out to take the fruit which is forbidden by the Lord, instantly the ecological balance is upset and nature begins to groan [14:14].

Thus it can be seen that an effective challenge to the orthodox anthropocentrism of the Christian view of nature can begin with at least one of the Creation narratives. But that is only a beginning. Anthropocentrism for its part relies on more than the Creation narratives for its biblical support. It points out that God made a specific covenant with man, and that his activity is in the historical life of a specific people, culminating in his Incarnation among those people. The prophets who served before his coming emphasized social righteousness, the proper behavior between man and man. The Incarnation itself was God as man, and not as some other creature or in some other form of expression. In addition, it could be pointed out that nature not subject to man's control — the wilderness — was where the erring children of Israel had to wander and suffer and where Christ was tempted. Finally, it could be noted that a commanding figure of the Kingdom come is the New Jerusalem, the city, which is the unique expression of man over against nature.

Yet with all this, the fact remains that the biocentric theme is clearly discernible throughout the scriptures, and its presence legitimizes those who speak from such a point of view. George H. Williams presents a kind of compendium of the biblical evidence calling for a biocentric perspective. Relative to the Creation narratives he mentions that, "Man was placed in the midst of Paradise as a steward to give names to and bewonder the teeming multitudes of forms that had before him issued from the hands of the Creator." He then goes on to point out that,

> Noah was instructed by God to preserve from universal destruction two or seven of every kind of beast and bird, both clean and unclean, that is, without due regard to their eventual utility to man. After the Flood and the legitimation of the eating of meat, the prophets could still look forward to the restitution of peace within the animal kingdom and of harmony between man and beast. One of them, Hosea (2:20), even foresaw God entering a covenant with the beasts of the field, the birds of the air, and the reptiles on the ground in order to secure the peace of the elect. Job (40:15) in understandably self-centered wretchedness was reminded by God of the comfort to be gained from perspective: "Behold now the hippopotamus which I made with thee." Jesus said that the heavenly Father regards the lily of the field and the sparrow that falls. Paul (Romans 8:22) thought of the whole creation as in some obscure way groaning together with man in pain until the redemption. The newly-discovered *Gospel According to Thomas* preserves a gospel of all creatures (1:4, 77–79) alongside the familiar gospel to all creatures (Mark 16:15) [26:x].

To this could be added the testimony of the psalmist concerning the care of the creatures by God (Psalm 104) as well as the fact that the wilderness does not always elicit a negative response in scripture. It was in the wilderness that the Decalogue was said to have been delivered (wilderness of the Sinai Peninsula), it was there that Elijah met God, and it was the wilderness which served as the "base of operations" for John the Baptist.

Thus it can be seen that the "biocentrist" need make no apology for his broader view, for imbedded in the sacred writings are large amounts of supporting evidence for his view — for those who have eyes to see it.

As to the numinous consciousness of Eiseley, here, too, it is not difficult to marshall support, and with evidence not from exotic but from "mainline" sources out of biblical and church history. In these we see none of the "desacralizing" tendency which has come to be so accepted.

So Eric Rust reminds us that the Hebrew mind viewed "wonders" (a possible translation of *niphla'ah* and *pele*, which can also be rendered "miracles") as events concerning a spectrum which to the modern man would inappropriately cover very ordinary happenings.

> The extraordinary event was indeed just as natural as the ordinary, since all were alike the direct manifestations of the divine creative power. Hence it is not surprising to find the Old Testament classifying very ordinary phenomena as miracles. For the coming of the autumn rains, and man's supply of daily bread, could be just as miraculous as those more abnormal events that the Medieval Church associated with its saints. The Psalmist finds a wonder in the structure of his own body [Psalm 139:14–16], and Job can declare that among the marvellous things without number which God does is the sending of rain upon the earth [Job 5:10] [21:81–82].

This whole viewpoint carried over into what we see recorded in the New Testament. Jesus pointed to the activity of God in relation to sparrows, lilies of the field, rain that fell on good and bad alike, and seeds sown in a field — ordinary events in everyone's view. Yet by the same activity he also is attested to have healed and otherwise acted in an extraordinary way, a "miraculous" way as a modern person would consider it. Yet if Christ is a focus of faith, a unique manifestation of God, then "ordinary" and "extraordinary" cannot be sharply separated. One can say that to Christ all things were wondrous (and this is the better description) or all things were ordinary, but stringent separation of events and processes was not in his apperception.

This "non-separation" mentality was also present in the Reformers. They saw God manifest in all the operations of nature and therefore viewed the "miraculous" very differently from many modern men, including many modern theologians. Calvin, as an example, could say of the "sign" of the rainbow:

> . . . if any philosophaster [sic], to deride the simplicity of our faith, shall contend that the variety of colours [of the rainbow] arises naturally from the rays reflected by the opposite cloud, let us admit the fact, but, at the same time deride his stupidity in not recognizing God as the Lord and governor of nature, who, at his pleasure, makes all the elements subservient to his glory. If he had impressed memorials of this description on the sun, the stars, the earth, and stones, they would all have been to us as sacraments [3:IV/XIV, 18].

Elsewhere Calvin points to the important analogical value of nature for the Christian faith, suggesting that attention to the activity of God in the former would help to affirm tenets in the latter. He said, "Nor would the thing [the Resurrection] be so difficult to belief were we as attentive as we ought to be of the wonders which meet our eye in every quarter of the world" [3:III/XXV, 4]. And, finally, commenting on Revelation 5:13 where "every creature" is seen praising the victorious Lamb, Calvin says, "It is absolutely certain that both irrational and inanimate creatures are [here] comprehended. All, then, which is affirmed is that every point of the universe, from the highest pinnacle of heaven to the very center of the earth, each in its own way, proclaims the glory of the Creator" [3:III/V, 8].

Today this kind of awareness is continued by a man such as Loren Eiseley. Certainly he is not as specifically religious as those mentioned above, and yet he sees the whole of nature in a way which can only be called religious. All life is wondrous to his way of thinking, as with the Hebrew, Christ, and Calvin. One objection that might have been raised about those cited in support of the numinous consciousness, that they all come from prescientific eras, is negated by the fact that the modern advocate, or better, possessor of such a consciousness is himself a scientist. This points to a deep irony in our modern day; for we find a "secular" scientist expressing a type of religious consciousness which influential theologians and other religious thinkers are inclined to dismiss. It is Eiseley for whom the biblical bush burns, while, say, for a Cox the light has been extinguished.

Noting this reversal of roles, the question is whether the influence of those for whom the light has gone out will prevail, and thus eliminate all possibility of an awareness of the numinous in those who are capable of response. Certainly in the kind of patterns of control one finds in Chardin, Richardson, and Cox the possibility of a numinous experience from nature will be practically nil. I, for one, would hold that to underwrite activities that would close off a channel of religious awareness is a spiritual outrage, comparable to a destruction of foodstuffs which would otherwise nurture a man physically. Somehow there must be a way whereby the separation of man and nature, so long dominant in the Christian world (though an important and countervailing minor theme within Christianity has been illustrated), can be overcome, both for the sake of man and for the sake of the rest of the natural order.

OVERCOMING SEPARATION FROM NATURE

For a suggestion on how to overcome the man-nature separation, I would turn, paradoxically, to the theological offerings of one of those whom I have characterized as supporting such a separation. Herbert Richardson writes that, "Theology must develop a conception of God which can undergird the primary realities of the cybernetics world, viz., systems." Then he adds: "And ethics must reorient its work in terms of these systems and focus on the problem of control . . . the God of a sociotechnic intellectus [context of meaning] must be reconceived as the unity of the manifold systems of the world" [18:23]. He mentions the fact that such a conception has already been developed by American theologians and philosophers such as Edwards, Emerson, Royce, and H. R. Niebuhr, and all that is required is the application of what is already at hand.

We might look at one of those whom Richardson mentions. H. R. Niebuhr, when talking about the effect of unity in God, notes that as he alone is considered holy a kind of Puritan iconoclasm arises, casting doubts on special and holy days, places, and so forth. However, he goes on to add that this phenomenon has an accompanying effect:

> The counterpart of this secularization . . . is the sanctification of all things. Now every day is the day that the Lord has made; every nation is a holy people called by him into existence in its place and time and to his glory; every person is sacred, made in his image and likeness; *every living thing, on earth, in the heavens, and in the waters, is his creation and points in its existence toward him; the whole earth is filled with his glory* [15:53–54, italics added].

These words are in perfect accord with those cited earlier from Calvin. Niebuhr says that everything created takes on significance; all things that make up the manifold systems of the world are related in God. Now the very critical question is: what are the manifold systems of the world? *All* the systems of the world are the manifold systems, and not just the "encompassing system of social relations" to which Richardson narrows his perspective after having called for the new orientation. The natural systems should be included in the calculus as well as social, economic, political, and formal religious systems of the world.

With natural systems included in the overall consideration, thus correcting Richardson's oversight, the theologian's suggestion of viewing God as the unity of the various systems as well as focusing on control becomes especially valuable. For now God may be seen as present not only in the affairs of men, but also in the postures of all other forms of life and Creation. The immanence of God in nature, so long suppressed by the dominant

Christian view and especially by neo-orthodox theologians and their present successors, can re-emerge, and the numinous consciousness of a man like Eiseley can now be theologically explained rather than being ignored or explained away. Also, control takes on a much more sophisticated meaning once the natural order is included. Where previously control has meant sheer subjugation of the given systems, now it will take on a symbiotic connotation, thus supporting the dictum of Francis Bacon which has been called the first principle of ecology: "We cannot command nature except by obeying her" [1:170].

Interpreting this last dictum in a specifically theological way, we may say that proper control is that which is in accord with God and, conversely, improper control is that which opposes God. If God is the unity of the systems, including nature, and man violates the systems, especially the natural one, then it follows that man in his violation is in confrontation with God. Here we recall the statements of Eiseley which emphasized how the emergent man who tries to extricate himself from the web of life will be subject to dire repercussions. The theological interpretation of this is that whenever man, either because of ignorance or arrogance, lives too far out of balance with the natural order, he meets God, the author of that order as well as the immanent being in it, as the God of wrath and judgment. To be sure, this is repugnant to many in an age given over to the glorification of man, but it is an implication legitimately drawn from a comprehensive "systems" theology.

As a result of the espousal of such a view, there comes the rejection of the completely man-dominated prognoses offered by Richardson and the other "anthropocentrists." What on first glance may appear as thrilling expressions of man's progress and control now are seen in a completely different way. Now they appear as patterns which lead to a baleful confrontation with God and to the abrogation of the integrity of the natural order, both in and of itself and as a means of numinous consciousness to man. In their stead arises the demand for a new view. In this view the emerging emphases are upon restraint, an appreciation of life in its full diversity, the maintenance of harmony between the various life forms and, most important, upon the preservation of large interstices of untrammeled nature for its own sake, and in order that man may still realize the workings and wonders of God.

REFERENCES

1. Bacon, Francis: quoted in Peter Farb: *Ecology* (*Life* Nature Library, Time, Inc, New York, New York) 1963.
2. Borgstrom, Georg: *The Hungry Planet* (Collier Books, The Macmillan Co, New York, New York) 1967.
3. Calvin, John: Institutes of the Christian Religion, Henry Beveridge, translator (Wm B Eerdmans Co, Grand Rapids, Michigan) 1957.
4. Chardin, Teilhard de: *The Phenomenon of Man*, Bernard Wall, translator (Harper Torchbooks, Harper & Row, New York, New York) 2nd ed, 1965.
5. *The Christian Century*, vol 85, no 3, Jan 17, 1968, p 69, editorial.
6. Commoner, Barry: *Science and Survival* (The Viking Press, New York, New York) 1967.
7. Cox, Harvey: *On Not Leaving It to the Snake* (The Macmillan Co, New York, New York) 1967.
8. Cox, Harvey: *The Secular City* (The Macmillan Co, New York, New York) 1965.
9. Eiseley, Loren: *The Firmament of Time* (Atheneum Publishers, New York, New York) 1967.
10. Eiseley, Loren: from The House We Live In, television program broadcast in Philadelphia, Pennsylvania, Feb 5, 1961.
11. Eiseley, Loren: *The Immense Journey* (Vintage Books, Random House, Inc, New York, New York) 1957.
12. Gates, Donald M: in *The New York Times*, Mar 20, 1968, p 14.
13. Harrington, Joseph J: data taken from a lecture at the School of Public Health, Harvard University, Boston, Massachusetts, Sept 29, 1967.

14. Moule, C F D: *Man and Nature in the New Testament* (The Fortress Press, Philadelphia, Pennsylvania) 1967.

15. Niebuhr, H R: *Radical Monotheism and Western Civilization* (University of Nebraska Press, Lincoln, Nebraska) 1960.

16. Rad, Gerhard von: *Genesis: A Commentary*, John H Marks, translator (The Westminster Press, Philadelphia, Pennsylvania) 1961.

17. *Restoring the Quality of Our Environment: Report of the Environmental Pollution Panel, President's Science Advisory Committee* (U.S. Government Printing Office, Washington, D.C.) 1965.

18. Richardson, Herbert: *Toward an American Theology* (Harper & Row, New York, New York) 1967.

19. Rudd, R L: *Pesticides in the Living Landscape* (University of Wisconsin Press, Madison, Wisconsin) 1964.

20. Ruskin, John: quoted in Rudolf Otto: *The Idea of the Holy*, John W Harvey, translator (Oxford University Press, New York, New York) 1958.

21. Rust, Eric C: *Nature and Man in Biblical Thought* (Lutterworth Press, London, England) 1953.

22. Sears, Paul B: Utopia and the Living Landscape, *Daedalus*, Spring 1965, p 484.

23. Task Force on Environmental Health and Related Problems: *Strategy for a Livable Environment* (U.S. Government Printing Office, Washington, D.C.) 1967.

24. Thomas, Harold A, jr: lecture at the School of Public Health, Harvard University, Boston, Massachusetts, Oct 6, 1967.

25. White, Lynn, jr: The Historical Roots of the Ecologic Crisis, *Science*, vol 155, no 3767, Mar 10, 1967, p 1205.

26. Williams, George H: *Wilderness and Paradise in Christian Thought* (Harper & Bros, New York, New York) 1962.

27. World Population Data Sheet (Population Reference Bureau, Washington, D.C.) Mar 1968.

NOTES ON CONTRIBUTORS

HENRY K. BEECHER, M.D., is anesthetist-in-chief at the Massachusetts General Hospital in Boston, Massachusetts, and Dorr Professor of Research in Anesthesia at Harvard University. He has written many articles for professional medical journals and the forthcoming *Research and the Individual: Human Experimentation*.

DANIEL CALLAHAN, former managing editor of *Commonweal*, is currently on a grant from the Population Council and the Ford Foundation to complete a book on abortion. Most recently he edited *The Catholic Case for Contraception* (1969).

ARTHUR J. DYCK is assistant professor of social ethics at Harvard Divinity School and a member of the Harvard Center for Population Studies.

FREDERICK ELDER is senior minister of the Faith Presbyterian Church in Minnetonka, Minnesota. His essay in this volume is based on a master's thesis at the Harvard Divinity School completed in 1968.

JOSEPH FLETCHER is Robert Treat Paine Professor of Social Ethics at the Episcopal Theological School in Cambridge, Massachusetts. His many writings include *Situation Ethics* (1966), *Moral Responsibility* (1967), and with Harvey Cox, *The Situation Ethics Debate* (1968).

JAMES M. GUSTAFSON is professor of Christian studies at Yale University. In 1968 he published *Christ and the Moral Life* and with James T. Laney edited *On Being Responsible: Issues in Personal Ethics*.

M. H. PAPPWORTH, M.D., is a member of Britain's Royal College of Physicians and the author of *Human Guinea Pigs: Experimentation on Man* (1967).

JULIAN R. PLEASANTS is assistant professor of microbiology at the University of Notre Dame in Indiana. He has written many essays on moral questions in science and on the biology of germfree animals.

RALPH B. POTTER, JR., is assistant professor of social ethics at the Harvard Divinity School and a member of the Harvard Center for Population Studies.

PAUL RAMSEY is Harrington Spear Paine Professor of Religion at Princeton University. During 1968–69 he is Joseph P. Kennedy, Jr., Foundation Visiting Professor of Genetic Ethics at Georgetown Medical School. His many writings include *Deeds and Rules in Christian Ethics* (1967) and *The Just War: Force and Political Responsibility* (1968).

HERBERT W. RICHARDSON is associate professor of theology at St. Michael's College of the University of Toronto. He is the author of *Toward an American Theology* (1967).

INDEX

Index